VALIDATION

VALIDATION

How the Skill Set That Revolutionized
Psychology Will Transform Your Relationships,
Increase Your Influence, and Change Your Life

CAROLINE FLECK, PhD

AVERY

an imprint of Penguin Random House

New York

an imprint of Penguin Random House LLC
penguinrandomhouse.com

Most Avery books are available at special quantity discounts for bulk purchase for sales promotions, premiums, fund-raising, and educational needs. Special books or book excerpts also can be created to fit specific needs. For details, write SpecialMarkets@penguinrandomhouse.com.

Library of Congress Cataloging-in-Publication Data

Names: Fleck, Caroline, author.
Title: Validation: How the Skill Set That Revolutionized Psychology
    Will Transform Your Relationships, Increase Your Influence, and
    Change Your Life / Caroline Fleck, PhD.
Description: New York: Avery, an imprint of Penguin Random House, [2025] |
    Includes index.
Identifiers: LCCN 2024005229 (print) | LCCN 2024005230 (ebook) |
    ISBN 9780593541210 (hardcover) | ISBN 9780593541234 (epub)
Subjects: LCSH: Dialectical behavior therapy. | Validation therapy.
Classification: LCC RC489.D48 F54 2025 (print) | LCC RC489.D48 (ebook) |
    DDC 616.89/142—dc23/eng/20240327
    LC record available at https://lccn.loc.gov/2024005229
    LC ebook record available at https://lccn.loc.gov/2024005230

Printed in the United States of America
1st Printing

Book design by Angie Boutin

To Havana: "When you came into the world,
you cried and it broke my heart."

CONTENTS

Introduction   *1*

PART 1
WHAT AND WHY

CHAPTER 1   Validation—Psychology's Best-Kept Secret   *9*

CHAPTER 2   A Cure for All—Why You Should Drop
Everything and Learn to Validate   *23*

CHAPTER 3   What It Means to Be Seen—Validation Defined   *39*

CHAPTER 4   Validation and the Art of Suffering—One Last
Reason to Drop Everything and Learn to Validate   *55*

PART 2
HOW

CHAPTER 5   The Validation Ladder—Eight Steps to Seeing
and Being Seen   *71*

CHAPTER 6   Attend—the Game All Good Listeners Play   *81*

CHAPTER 7   Copy—How to Connect with Anyone   *99*

CHAPTER 8   Contextualize—Solving for Why   *113*

CHAPTER 9   Equalize—The "Anyone in Your Shoes Would
Do the Same" Skill   *125*

CHAPTER 10   Propose—How to Read Minds   *141*

CHAPTER 11   Take Action—When Words Aren't Enough   *157*

CHAPTER 12   Emote—My Advice for Jimmy Kimmel   *173*

CHAPTER 13   Disclose—The Power of Me, Too   *189*

PART 3

WHERE CHANGE COMES IN

CHAPTER 14   Ch, Ch, Ch, Changes—Behavioral Change Strategies   *205*

CHAPTER 15   Raising Emotionally Intelligent Children—
              Validation and Parenting   *215*

CHAPTER 16   The Universal Love Language—
              Validation in Intimate Relationships   *229*

CHAPTER 17   Validate Like a Boss—Validation at Work   *239*

CHAPTER 18   Everybody Hurts—Self-Validation   *251*

              Epilogue   *269*

Appendix   *275*

Acknowledgments   *277*

Notes   *281*

Index   *299*

NOTE

The word *patient* implies a degree of passivity that is at odds with the collaborative relationship I try to foster in my therapy practice. For this reason, I, like many therapists before me, refer to those I treat as "clients." Also, I used pseudonyms for the clients I reference in this book, so if you run into someone named Dev who matches the description of the client I describe in chapter 2, it's not her.

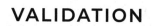

VALIDATION

INTRODUCTION

I've always been a sensitive person. When I was younger, this seemed like a blessing. People were drawn to me. I have a smattering of flashbulb memories from childhood of folks confiding their deepest insecurities and secrets in me as though they were talking to themselves in a mirror. Not just kids, but adults, too. I remember in third grade when my friend Jenny's mom told me that her husband was having an affair. One minute I'm waiting for Jenny to return home from dance practice so we could go to her basement and pretend the floor was lava; the next, I'm crouched next to her mom on the floor, trying to ignore the two liters of Pepsi she'd accidentally knocked over. The details of her unraveling marriage seemed to just pour out of her, almost uncontrollably, punctuated by deep moans. I don't remember a word she said to me; I imagine most of it was over my head. But I never forgot the look on her face: wild eyes and cheeks smeared with tears and spit. She was describing something I knew nothing about, but still, I tried to attune to her. "This is awful," I said as the soda pooled at my feet. "It's like being born and dying at the same time." I was nine years old; what did I know about divorce or "starting over"?! Despite the fact that I didn't know what the hell I was talking about, my words seemed to resonate with her.

I didn't always succeed in saying or doing the right thing in moments like these. I don't ever recall making the situation worse, but there were plenty of times when I failed to intuit what others were feeling or needing. When I did manage to connect, though, the experience was electric. I felt worthy, helpful, and kind.

Unfortunately, as I got older, my sensitivity became more of a curse. Rather than drawing people to me, it began to have the opposite effect—it distanced me from them. I seemed to get hurt more easily than others, and by my teens, I was taking much longer than my friends to recover from the emotional sunburns of adolescence. I began to feel alone and vulnerable much of the time. The technical name for what I experienced is Queen Elsa of Arendelle syndrome. Just kidding, it's major depressive disorder. I was diagnosed at age sixteen and spent more than a decade battling the debilitating symptoms. I was withdrawn and guarded for much of this time. But every now and then, I'd try to rediscover those magical connections I'd chased as a child. And every now and then, I'd be rewarded with the exquisite experience of connecting with someone as though they were myself.

Those moments of connection offered brief reprieves from the suffering that had come to define me. The only other escape I found was in books and studying. As an undergraduate, I spent many nights cocooned in the library's study rooms behind a fortress of articles and papers that seemed to protect me from myself. By senior year, I'd decided to pursue a doctorate in clinical psychology, knowing it would buy me many more years of assignments in which to hide. I also hoped that I might one day learn how to channel my sensitivity in ways that helped others more and hurt me less. The power in my emotions was apparent; if only I could learn how to harness it. Remarkably, there came a time when I learned to do just that.

I won't go so far as to say, "I'll never forget the day" I learned about validation because, like most people, I forget most of most days. But I do vividly remember a deep purple PowerPoint slide with the heading "Acceptance Strategies: Validation," and I distinctly remember listening to the dynamic lecture and thinking, "Why don't they teach this in grade schools?!"

Learning about validation and the skills used to communicate it felt like discovering pieces of a puzzle I'd not realized were missing. I'm talking, like, *corner* pieces. I had immediate insight into how the sensitivity that plagued me could become a buoy for those around me. The "magic" I'd chased all my life was revealed to be a simple method anyone could master. The more I practiced validating, the better I got at it, and the more connected I felt to myself and others. Over time, my perspective on my emotions changed, as did my relationship with them. **Validation transformed my sensitivity from a weakness I felt desperate to protect into a superpower I could use to help others.**

I want to state clearly that practicing validation did not single-handedly cure me of depression, nor am I aware of any data to suggest it would. What I do know, through personal experience and extensive research, is that validation has a profound effect on relationships and your ability to affect change within them. This goes for your relationships with others *and* with yourself. The positive changes you can expect from validation are diverse but generally fall into one of five categories:

1. **Improved relationships:** Validation affects how relationships *feel*. Increased intimacy, camaraderie, trust, and psychological safety are to be expected after you've succeeded in deeply validating someone's experience. Changing how people feel inevitably affects how they behave. If you've increased trust and safety through validation, you can expect to see more transparency and engagement in the relationship.

2. **Decreased conflict:** Incorporating validation into difficult conversations keeps them from going in circles or descending into arguments. People tend to use force or "attack" when they believe they can't get their point across otherwise. Similarly, folks become defensive when they feel the need to defend a position that isn't being respected. A validating response leaves nothing to attack, much less anything to defend against.

3. **Increased influence:** It's hard to solve a problem or convince people of something if they think you don't understand where they're coming from. Validating people helps

you not only communicate understanding but cultivate it. As a result, folks are more likely to talk *and* listen to you.

4. **Increased ability to drive behavior change:** Validation is free to provide, everyone wants it, and unlike candy, people don't get sick of it. These attributes make validation a powerful reinforcement that can drive all sorts of behavioral changes, like getting someone to exercise and possibly even reducing opioid use.[1]

5. **Increased self-compassion:** Validating others transforms how we relate to them and to ourselves. Just as sitting alone in meditation improves our connection with others, connecting with others via validation improves our relationship with ourselves. These benefits can be further enhanced through the practice of self-validation described later in the book.

In the decade or so since learning validation skills, I've made it my mission to share them with as many people as possible. During this time, I've seen them single-handedly salvage marriages, redefine parent-child dynamics, and even save lives. (More on that later.) Validation is often the first thing I teach in therapy, parenting workshops, and corporate trainings. When a Big Five tech company asked me to design a twelve-week interpersonal effectiveness course for a hundred employees, I devoted a third of it to validation. Outcomes from this class exceeded corporate leaders' expectations; the most frequent feedback we received was a request for books on validation.

You don't need to be a sensitive person or an "empath" to develop the validation skills that will allow you to achieve these changes. The fact that I stumbled upon the magic of validation at a young age meant I had a knack for it, but raw talent is not a prerequisite for developing these skills. Ironically, I've found that folks who are innately more sensitive and take to these skills naturally are less inclined to practice and, therefore, *less* likely to master them. (I'll explain why later.) Emotional sensitivity is an advantage, that's for sure, but without practice, that advantage will take you only so far.

In the coming pages, I'll show you how to consistently achieve those magical connections I spent so much of my life chasing and how to translate them into meaningful changes. In organizing the content for this book, I relied heavily on principles of learning like repetition and modeling to ensure you get the most out of any effort you put in. Still, there's no getting around the fact that you will need to do more than read this book to achieve the transformations it promises. As with any language, studying it in a book will get you only so far. To become a fluent speaker, you must practice speaking.

PART 1

WHAT AND WHY

CHAPTER 1

VALIDATION—PSYCHOLOGY'S BEST-KEPT SECRET

In a gentle way, you can shake the world.
—COMMONLY ATTRIBUTED TO MAHATMA GANDHI

I was a twenty-seven-year-old doctoral student in clinical psychology sitting across from a twenty-two-year-old man who had just told me, matter-of-factly, that he was thinking about killing himself that evening. Behind him was a camera, focused on me, and a monitor. The sentence "Always assess suicidality at the START!" appeared on the monitor. My eyes flicked to the clock. I was in the last five minutes of an hour-long session. Down the hall, my pixelated face was projected on a screen in front of a classroom of ten other trainees and my clinical instructor, who was typing his feedback to me in real time.

I quickly ran through a series of questions to assess my client's risk: Did he have access to lethal means? Had he thought through a plan? etc. His risk, I determined, was moderate. He disclosed that he'd broken up with his boyfriend two nights ago. He hadn't mentioned it earlier because he did *not* want to talk about it. As the session was winding down, he'd started thinking about returning to the empty apartment that he had until recently shared with his partner. He said he didn't think he could tolerate another night on his own.

I knew what to do. I needed to help him use the skills he was developing to bring down his despair in our session and then discuss how he could use those same skills at home to get him through the night. But I had a problem. He didn't want to use any skills; he was convinced they wouldn't work. He also didn't want to talk about the breakup and he was irritated with me for asking him so many questions. He said he wished he hadn't said anything; he just wanted to go home.

If I didn't turn things around quickly, I'd have to consider hospitalizing him against his will, because he did not want to be admitted to the hospital. And if I hospitalized him, I risked losing him as a patient and souring him on the therapy he so desperately needed. I looked to the monitor for answers. It was blank. I started pulling out all the cognitive behavioral strategies I could think of. Positive reinforcement, Socratic questioning, negative reinforcement, modeling, begging (okay, that last one is not technically a strategy)—none of it worked. I looked at the clock and then at the monitor. To this day, I can still see the letters V-A-L-I-D-A-T-I-O-N appearing slowly on the screen. For a moment, I was confused. He explicitly said he didn't want to talk about the breakup. Then it hit me.

"This sucks," I said.

He looked up. More like he *glared* up, if that's a thing.

"You let your guard down for one second and are immediately attacked with questions from the overzealous graduate student you want to believe gives a shit but is most likely just doing what she's told."

I glanced at the monitor. The word *Good* appeared.

"And if that wasn't enough, the whole thing is being broadcast to a room full of people you've never met."

"I'm usually pretty good at tuning that out. Thanks for the reminder," he said . . . with a smile!

"I am, too, but right now, it's distracting me," I confided, and with that, I stood up, stepped over to the monitor, and turned it off. I then suggested we take a walk. We spent the next twenty minutes meandering through the gardens across from the cognitive behavioral treatment center. Our conversation was an extension of the one we'd had in the room, with me just trying to put myself in his shoes. I didn't attempt to talk him out of suicide or reduce his risk in any way. Instead, I focused on trying to connect with the experience of this person who desperately needed help but had learned not to trust anyone who offered it.

When we got back, we got to work. The session lasted more than two hours. In the end, I made the decision not to hospitalize him. This was the right call. He used the skills we practiced in session at home that night and got through it on his own. He got through the next night, too, and the one after that. It's been almost two decades since we worked together. He often sends me updates and photos from the "life worth living" he has built for himself. He's now a therapist, too, and an excellent one at that.

Convincing someone to cope with extreme pain rather than commit suicide is an admittedly high-stakes example of influencing someone's behavior. But the strategies that work in delicate situations like these are equally effective, if not more so, in less extreme scenarios. I always say that the only difference between influencing people in therapy and influencing them outside of it is that the former is often more challenging. You can imagine how much harder it would be to compel someone to exercise regularly if they were suffering from crippling depression and had lost the motivation to do even their favorite activities. It's true that experts in clinical psychology know the *types* of changes that are likely to improve various mental health symptoms and disorders,* but the strategies they use to foster change apply to people generally, not just those with mental illness.[1]

Psychologists obviously aren't the only ones interested in changing how people think or behave. We all spend an excessive amount of time trying to get people to listen to us, and despite our best efforts, we often fail. I'd be willing to bet that, right now, there's at least one person in your life you're struggling to influence. Perhaps

---

* Regular exercise, by the way, is as effective as antidepressants at treating depression. (James A. Blumenthal et al., "Exercise and Pharmacotherapy in the Treatment of Major Depressive Disorder," *Psychosomatic Medicine* 69, no. 7 [September 1, 2007]: 587–96, https://doi.org/10.1097/psy.0b013e318148c19a.)

someone at home—your kid, partner, or parent. Or someone at your job—a manager or a colleague. You want them to work more, work less, stop talking about work, respond to your messages, quit messaging you, learn how to use Messenger . . . the ways in which we want the people around us to change are infinite.

Not surprisingly, change is a billion-dollar industry. Every year, we flock to workshops, books, and retreats that promise to help us change the behavior of others or improve our relationships with them. These resources are usually focused on specific types of dynamics or problems—"How to Lead So People Will Listen" or "How to Parent Oppositional Children," for example. Their aim, however, is essentially the same—to help you influence behavior.

There's a lot of pseudoscience and straight-up bullshit out there on how to influence people, but there's also a surprising amount of credible information. Scientifically proven *change strategies* like positive reinforcement have become increasingly commonplace. These techniques, which have been used for decades in cognitive behavioral therapies, are now the hallmarks of successful programs for issues ranging from potty training to job retention. (Let's all pause for a second to appreciate that potty training and job retention can be achieved using similar methods.)

It makes sense that people would be interested in the scientific approaches psychologists use to influence behavior, particularly in difficult situations. Like I said, we all have people around us who seem immune to influence, and the thought that we might actually be able to get through to them is exciting. What's harder to understand is why everyone keeps rehashing a handful of behavioral strategies from more than seventy years ago without mentioning any of the more recent research on how to enhance them. This BLOWS. MY. MIND. Our insights on how to affect human behavior didn't end with B. F. Skinner.* That's where they began!

The early findings from behavioral research are still relevant.

---

* B. F. Skinner is considered the father of behaviorism. His claim to fame was his work on operant conditioning, which introduced the concepts of reinforcements and punishments.

Anyone who has ever trained a dog knows that positively reinforcing them with a treat goes a long way toward getting them to sit
or shake on command. And it's well established that this early
research on behaviorism doesn't apply only to animals; just
the thought of advancing deeper into a game is enough to compel
some people to hole up in internet cafés for days on end. What
we've learned in the years since Skinner, though, is that when
people are resistant to changing their ways, it's not enough to know
how to apply basic principles of change. You also need to know how
to demonstrate acceptance.

WHY CHANGE REQUIRES ACCEPTANCE

Clinical psychologists have been researching the relationship
between acceptance and behaviorism since the early 1990s, when
Dr. Marsha Linehan introduced a new type of treatment called Dialectical Behavior Therapy (DBT). Linehan's treatment sent shock-
waves through the field, not only because it showed that acceptance
is a catalyst for change but also because it proved capable of doing
what no other therapy in the history of time had managed to do:
reliably reduce self-harm and suicidal behavior in people with
these conditions.[2]

In the landscape of modern psychology, "acceptance" means
acknowledging the reality of a situation without judging or trying
to change it. Based on this definition, acceptance and change are
literally incompatible. But as a young researcher who was struggling to treat suicidal clients using traditional behavioral strategies, Linehan began to think that acceptance and change might be
two sides of the same coin. She theorized that overemphasizing
change could cause people to become resistant to it. Imagine how
that session I described at the beginning of the chapter would have
gone if I'd kept pushing my client to use his skills. Linehan also
suspected that certain mental health problems are caused by pervasive invalidation—frequent messages from the environment that
a person or their emotions are unacceptable. If you compare the

suicide rates of those in the LGBTQIA+ community to those outside of it, you can see the merit of this perspective.[3]

Linehan thought that if people felt genuinely accepted, they might be more receptive to change. To test her hypothesis, she developed a new type of therapy—DBT—that had therapists use their trusted behavioral change strategies alongside a set of acceptance strategies she developed. The latter consisted primarily of validation skills designed to help therapists communicate acceptance as well as some skills to help clients accept themselves and their circumstances. The term *acceptance strategies* describes this collection of therapist and client skills, and validation is chief among them. In Linehan's words, "It would be difficult to overestimate the importance of validation in DBT."[4] In my words, validation is what Justin Timberlake was to *NSYNC or what Beyoncé was to Destiny's Child. The other acceptance strategies have their place in the ensemble, but they pale in comparison to validation.

Following DBT's success, a new wave of therapies based on the model of acceptance and change swept the field. Collectively, these therapies have proven effective in reducing a wide range of mental health problems and are now the gold standard for treating conditions like recurrent depression[5] and borderline personality disorder,[6] which confounded psychologists for generations.

During the last few decades, as mental health topics have become less taboo, acceptance strategies have started making their way into the mainstream. Just last year, I saw a video[7] of Lady Gaga teaching Oprah "radical acceptance," the DBT skill she claims transformed her life by helping her cope with chronic pain.[8] As a psychologist, there are few things I love more than popping into a bookstore to find that an acceptance strategy I've only ever seen in treatment manuals is the title of a new bestseller. With scientific approaches to change and acceptance now both in high demand, you'd expect those uber-powerful validation skills to be on everybody's radar. But they're not.

As a buzzword, *validation* has undoubtedly been trending. At some point, we all seem to have absorbed the message that it's good for relationships. There just isn't a ton of information on what it means, much less how to practice it. The validation skills that have proven to help people communicate acceptance are not common knowledge. As for the discovery that validation is an agent for change, that, too, is a secret to most. Alas, although many acceptance strategies have entered the cultural zeitgeist, DBT's groundbreaking validation skills remain outside of it.

I don't mean to suggest that other acceptance skills you may have heard about, like radical acceptance, aren't transformative. They are! Practicing them regularly will affect how you relate to yourself and, arguably, how others relate to you over time. But they won't make you immediately more effective at influencing someone's behavior or increase the odds that they'll take your advice. A handful of validation skills, however, can do just that. **Validating will improve your ability to influence behavior, period. Failing to validate people will often render you totally ineffective, and in some scenarios, it will actually damage the person or relationship you hope to affect.**

Importantly, this connection between validation and change applies to yourself as much as it does to others—knowing how to self-validate will improve your relationship with yourself and the likelihood that you'll actually succeed in making the changes you want to make. Given DBT's success and the popularity of many of the skills and concepts it introduced, it's weird that its secret ingredient—validation—remains relatively unknown. Having spent years trying to get to the bottom of what's going on here, I've concluded that validation suffers from three major problems:

1. Validation means different things to different people.
2. Validation skills have been reserved for treating mental illness.
3. Validation skills are everywhere and nowhere.

These three problems explain why validation remains psychology's best-kept secret. In an effort to blow the lid off this secret, I'll *quickly* discuss each problem next and provide solutions to remedy them. **Understanding the issues associated with validation is the first step toward understanding the concept itself.**

PROBLEM #1: VALIDATION MEANS DIFFERENT THINGS TO DIFFERENT PEOPLE

If you're unclear on what validation means, you're not alone. Definitions of the term vary widely. The concept of "mindfulness" suffered from a similar problem when it first started to make waves in psychology following the success of Mindfulness-Based Stress Reduction (MBSR).[9] MBSR is an eight-week class that teaches mindfulness to people with no previous training in meditation or Buddhism. By the early 1990s, researchers had shown that MBSR improved conditions as diverse as chronic pain[10] and anxiety,[11] but the general public remained largely confused by the concept of mindfulness. Is it a religion? A mind state? A café in Los Angeles? Like validation, few could agree on what it meant, much less how to practice it.

Finally, in 1994, Jon Kabat-Zinn, PhD, the psychologist who developed MBSR, wrote a book on mindfulness for a nonacademic audience titled *Wherever You Go, There You Are.* In it, he defined mindfulness as "the awareness that arises from paying attention, on purpose, in the present moment and non-judgmentally."[12] Baking the directions for practicing mindfulness into the definition made the concept immediately more accessible, and the secular language distanced the term from the spiritual connotations of meditation. To this day, Kabat-Zinn's remains one of the most frequently cited definitions of mindfulness in the Western world.

Unlike mindfulness, which was associated with concepts like meditation and largely considered a cognitive process, validation is associated with terms like *praise* and considered the driving force behind why people use Instagram. According to Linehan, however, "Validation has nothing to do with social desirability and is not synonymous with praise."[13] The confusion surrounding validation is compounded by the fact that we've been warned never to seek it.

PUT SIMPLY, VALIDATION SHOWS THAT YOU'RE THERE, YOU GET IT, AND YOU CARE.

The message seems to be that validation is a good thing to bring to our relationships, but it's a needy and unhealthy thing to expect from them.

If the problem is that validation has come to mean different things to different people, then the obvious solution is to clearly define it. Easier said than done. I, for one, struggled for years to find a concise definition that resonated with my clients and mapped onto the skills I was teaching them. My understanding of validation came from the research literature, and these descriptions tended to be too jargony. It wasn't until I experimented with Kabat-Zinn's approach of leading with instruction that I landed on a definition that clicked with my clients and ultimately laid the foundation for my approach: **Validation: communication that one is *mindful*, *understands*, and *empathizes* with another person's experience, thereby accepting it as valid.** Put simply, validation shows that you're there, you get it, and you care.

The validation skills you'll learn in this book are tried-and-true techniques for communicating mindfulness, understanding, and empathy in ways that reflect acceptance.

PROBLEM # 2: VALIDATION SKILLS HAVE BEEN RESERVED FOR TREATING MENTAL ILLNESS

Clients in DBT learn many skills to help them manage emotions, become more mindful, increase interpersonal effectiveness, and cultivate acceptance. But the validation skills taught to therapists and instructions on how to master them were not originally offered to clients when DBT was introduced in the 1990s. Like therapists, those in DBT learned that validation is essential to building and maintaining relationships. They just weren't taught how to do it. At least, not until 2014, when Linehan updated the treatment manual and included validation skills among those taught to clients.[14] To this day, these skills are still often considered optional and may or may not be taught in DBT programs. Seeing as how validation skills have historically been reserved for therapists, it's not terribly surprising they've been slow to catch on.*

This leads me to my next point: Linehan was focused on helping people who were in hell get out of it, a laudable and career-consuming task. Unlike Kabat-Zinn, who defined mindfulness in a book targeting the general public, Linehan's approach to validation has been mostly confined to treatment manuals, clinical research articles, and the few handouts later developed for clients. Does this mean validation is effective only when used by therapists or people with mental illness? Nope. No. Nuh-uh. As you'll see in chapter 2, validation has been shown to decrease conflict, increase connection, and drive all sorts of behavioral changes, from motivating detainees to disclose credible information during interrogations to compelling teens to take their parents' advice. Does it mean those in the field need to do a better job of sharing this research and teaching these skills? Yes. Should they think more about how to translate them and demonstrate their broader utility? Hell, yeah!

This book is the culmination of the work I've done during the last decade to refine, reconceptualize, and expand DBT's validation skills so that anyone can use them to communicate understanding and build rapport across situations and relationships. In it, you will find answers to questions like "What should I say?" and

---

* The initial lack of emphasis on teaching validation to clients in DBT wasn't an oversight. Linehan spent decades refining her work on validation and piloting different ways of teaching it to clients. This type of meticulous research takes time but is par for the course when developing treatment protocols.

"How should I say it?" that so frequently stand between us and the people we hope to affect.

PROBLEM # 3: VALIDATION SKILLS ARE EVERYWHERE AND NOWHERE

It's true that validation skills have mainly been discussed in regard to therapy, but if you know what you're looking for, you'll find that these skills pop up all the time under different names. The problem is that they're rarely called "validation skills" or associated with the word *validation* at all. Instead, they tend to be presented as one-off solutions for specific relationship issues. For example, if you take a couples workshop, you're likely to learn the "speaker-listener" technique to help you better communicate with your partner.[15] If you read *Crucial Conversations* for work, you'll learn the "paraphrase skill" to help you effectively mitigate conflicts.[16] And if you're struggling to connect with your fourth-grader, you might be encouraged to practice "mirroring."[17] What might not be obvious to someone who isn't comparing these strategies side by side is that they all basically have you do the same thing— summarize or reflect what someone has said to demonstrate that you're listening and paying attention. They are all essentially variations of the same validation skill. I'll review this particular skill in part 2.

Because validation skills are rarely associated with the term *validation* and are constantly being rebranded as antidotes for very specific problems, it's difficult to recognize them for what they are. This difficulty is compounded by the fact that, as I've discussed, our general understanding of validation has been murky at best. As a result, it seems validation skills are both everywhere and nowhere.

Understanding what validation is and how to communicate it will help you identify validation skills, regardless of what they're called. Once you recognize that validation is what the situation calls for, you can use any of the skills in this book to achieve similar or better results. Because validation is everywhere and nowhere, mastering it is a bit like "seeing the matrix"—understanding how, why, and under what conditions it operates makes you infinitely more effective at influencing change.

LOOKING FORWARD

This book is divided into three parts. The chapters in this first part fully flesh out the concept of validation, review the remarkable outcomes associated with it, and briefly discuss how they came to be. Part 2 then introduces the Validation Ladder—the framework I've developed for teaching validation skills—and the never-before-published instructions on how to master them. Finally, part 3 shows you how to use these skills with standard behavioral change strategies like reinforcement and problem-solving to transform your life in the ways that matter most to you, from salvaging a marriage to silencing your inner critic. By the end of this book, you'll be equipped with everything you need to start experiencing the power of validation firsthand.

I focused a lot on DBT in this chapter, but I want to flag that I don't reference it much moving forward. The exception is in chapter 4, where I discuss the science and philosophy behind validation and how meeting Marsha Linehan challenged everything I thought I knew about validation—and multiple sclerosis, for that matter. For those looking to learn more about DBT, I highly recommend Linehan's memoir, *Building a Life Worth Living*.

Finally, I want to state clearly that this book will not teach you how to bend people to your will. It's true that validation unlocks the potential for change, but it does so through acceptance. Every single one of us wants to be seen and accepted for who we are. Meeting this need will incline people to listen to you. That's a fact. It will also inspire you to do better by them. As President Barack Obama said, "Learning to stand in somebody else's shoes, to see through their eyes, that's how peace begins. And it's up to you to make that happen."[18] Seeing through another person's eyes—bearing witness, understanding, and really caring about another person's experience—is easier said than done. It's not enough to want this or know that it's important; we must know how to do it. The skills and strategies included in this book are designed to do just that. They foster connection, resolution, and growth, but they demand it from you in return.

CHAPTER 2

A CURE FOR ALL—WHY YOU SHOULD DROP EVERYTHING AND LEARN TO VALIDATE

When the study began, nobody cared about empathy or attachment.
But the key to healthy aging is relationships, relationships, relationships.
—GEORGE VAILLANT, ON THE HARVARD STUDY OF ADULT DEVELOPMENT*

A few years back I began working with a woman, Dev, who was desperate to reconnect with her daughter, from whom she'd been estranged for several years. I can say without hesitation that Dev was one of the most gentle, incredible people I've ever had the pleasure of knowing. A recently retired cardiac surgeon, she donated more than half of her income every year to charities. When she wasn't working with Habitat for Humanity, she was fostering animals from local kill shelters. Dev was a soft-spoken force to be reckoned with, so it was hard to imagine how her relationship with her daughter, Kamia, could have deteriorated to the point of estrangement. I asked Dev to forward me the many texts and emails she'd sent Kamia in her efforts to reconnect. Dev's messages were

---

* The Harvard Study of Adult Development was a study conducted over the course of eighty years that set out to discover which factors (wealth, fame, relationships, etc.) have the biggest effect on human health and happiness. Spoiler alert: the answer is relationships. (Liz Mineo, "Over Nearly 80 Years, Harvard Study Has Been Showing How to Live a Healthy and Happy Life," *Harvard Gazette*, April 5, 2023, https://news .harvard.edu/gazette/story/2017/04/over-nearly-80-years-harvard-study-has-been -showing-how-to-live-a-healthy-and-happy-life.)

warm, upbeat, and positive—all qualities I'd observed in my own interactions with her. They were also invalidating. This is not what I would have expected from Dev, but it also didn't surprise me, given the issues they were having.

Kamia was nearing the end of her senior year of college. Although she loved school and was on a full scholarship, she suffered from chronic leukemia and had struggled throughout college. Dev hadn't spoken to her daughter since Thanksgiving of Kamia's sophomore year, when they had a heated fight, ostensibly over whether or not to see a movie. It ended with Kamia calling Dev a "self-righteous bitch who sucked all the joy out of life and replaced it with poison." In the years since, Kamia had been hospitalized twice following nights of heavy drinking, which Dev knew about only because she'd been contacted by the ER in the middle of the night. The hospitalizations would weigh on any parent, but they were particularly distressing for Dev, given Kamia's condition and their falling-out. She was eager to put the past behind them and attend to her highest priority, Kamia's health.

Not surprisingly, Dev's messages to her daughter following their estrangement were very focused on her disease. Dev would occasionally, kinda, sorta acknowledge the current state of their relationship: "I know it probably makes you cringe to see another note from your dear old mom . . ." But she was quick to minimize their issues and the emotions surrounding them: "All moms and daughters go through this type of thing. The sooner we can laugh about it, the better off we'll be." These platitudes were almost exclusively used to open or close a message, the bulk of which invariably focused on Kamia's health. "Here's an article I came across on how alcohol compromises immune functioning. 😷" or "I'm thinking of coming out in March to bring some leftover medical supplies and an updated EpiPen. I'm guessing yours expired like 4 years ago.😬" or my favorite, "I've scheduled a telehealth appointment for you with Dr. Jones. I know you didn't like her when you met back in high school, but she's one of the best hematologist-oncologists in the country. 🙏" Again, Kamia hadn't responded to a single one of her mom's messages in almost three years. Suffice it to say, she no-showed for the telehealth call. 😵

Dev agreed to take a break from messaging Kamia while she worked on developing the validation skills I share in this book. She focused on learning and practicing one skill a week until she knew them cold and could reliably use and identify them. When I was confident that she could "speak the language" of validation, I asked her to take a second look at the messages she'd shared with me when we first started working together. Dev said she could recall what she wrote, but I asked her to reread them anyway. She perused each message carefully, shaking her head slowly from left to right, wincing from time to time, and at one point biting her lip.

"Okay," she said, "I guess I didn't remember what I wrote. Turns out I'm a self-righteous bitch who sucks all the joy out of life and replaces it with poison."

Dev obviously wasn't a self-righteous bitch. At least, that was obvious to me. She was a loving, devoted mother who was showing up week after week in an effort to repair a relationship with a daughter who had hurt her deeply. Given their estrangement and Kamia's words, though, Dev was now struggling to see herself as anything other than a "bad parent." Addressing this belief was as critical to me as improving her communication with Kamia. **Self-invalidation is like a cancer—it spreads throughout the system, becoming increasingly difficult to contain.** It also operates like a cruel, self-fulfilling prophecy. Feelings of insecurity undermine a person's ability to be effective, which in turn reinforces their insecurity. In working to help Dev mend her relationship with Kamia, I focused equally on helping her validate herself. More on this later!

Progress on the relationship front was slow in the beginning. Dev focused first on acknowledging the current state of their relationship: "I shouldn't have made light of us not speaking. The truth is that it's heartbreaking, and I'm sorry we're in this place." Then we transitioned to having her validate the struggles and heartache of having a chronic medical condition, rather than intervening with medical supplies or doctors' appointments. After four weeks, Dev received her first response: "I love you, Mom. DON'T take that to mean I want you to fly out here." By the end of month three, they were exchanging messages regularly, and shortly after that, they began chatting on the phone. In time, they not only repaired their relationship, but also improved it. Every year since I've received a postcard from Dev at Thanksgiving with a picture of her and Kamia on location with Habitat for Humanity.

I opened this book by making some pretty bold claims about how mastering validation will transform your life. Specifically, I said that knowing how to validate people will help you do the following:

1. Improve relationships
2. Decrease conflict
3. Influence people
4. Drive change
5. Develop self-compassion

Stories like Dev's help illustrate my points, but an anecdote isn't a substitute for scientific evidence. I always find it disappointing, and suspicious, when people tout the remarkable effects of their approach without providing any data to substantiate their claims. I'm like, "Really? Your four-step plan will help me find love, lose weight, get promoted, and type faster? I'm loving the well-crafted stories, but could you share a study or two to assuage my doubts?" Rather than asking you to take me at my word, I want to share the research behind each of my five claims. I know, I know, research sounds super boring, but I promise, it won't be! Collectively, this science makes a compelling case for why you should drop everything and learn to validate. The data show that validation not only improves lives but can actually save them.

CLAIM #1: VALIDATION WILL IMPROVE YOUR RELATIONSHIPS

I know I just promised science, but I'm going to back into it by way of imagination. Try to think of something you might be hesitant to share with another person. It could be a secret you've never told anyone, a past transgression that evokes shame to this day, or a belief you doubt others would share. Next, visualize yourself sitting across from someone whose opinion you value, like your partner, parent, or friend, and telling them this information. Perhaps even say what you're thinking out loud—if you're alone—like you're talking to them. Now imagine this person responding in a way that makes you feel totally seen and accepted (i.e., validated). Visualize their facial expressions, and imagine what they might say to convey that they don't think any less of you. How do you suppose this experience would make you feel? Safe? Happy? Secure? Would you feel closer to this person and more inclined to trust them in the future? If you answered yes to any of these questions, you're not alone.

Validation improves relationships by transforming how they *feel*: it increases *trust, intimacy,* and *psychological safety.*[1]* Research has consistently shown validation to be among the strongest predictor of relational outcomes, ranging from commitment to quality, across various types of relationships.[2] It's basically like MDMA, except it's not harmful to the body. In fact, quite the opposite: by improving relationships, validation can affect a person's health and *life expectancy.* Having poor social relationships is associated with the same death rate as smoking fifteen cigarettes a day.[3] **Data show that a person's relationships can increase their probability**

---

* The studies cited are from the field of social psychology, where validation is referred to as Perceived Partner Responsiveness (PPR). PPR is defined as a response that registers as *understanding, validating,* and *caring* to the person receiving it. Their thing is close enough to my thing that I think it's safe to call it all the same thing. (Yan Ruan et al., "Can I Tell You How I Feel? Perceived Partner Responsiveness Encourages Emotional Expression," *Emotion* 20, no. 3 [April 1, 2020]: 2, https://doi.org/10.1037/emo0000650.)

of surviving by 50 percent.[4] I was serious when I said validation can save lives.

Importantly, validation packs a powerful punch regardless of whether we've shared anything vulnerable or even know the person who is validating us. In a clever study[5] that looked at the effects of validation on pain, researchers had participants hold a bucket of water at arm's length for as long as possible four times with a break in between each "pain trial." Unbeknownst to the participants, they were randomly put into one of two groups: those in the first group received validating responses from the experimenters in between each trial, and those in the second were given invalidating responses. Participants who received the validating statements reported more positive feelings and less worry compared to those in the invalidation group. They literally felt better. What's more, when asked if they'd be willing to participate in a fifth trial, those in the validation group were twice as likely to say yes. Let me repeat that: validation made people more likely to engage in another round of pain.

I don't know for certain how validation functioned to improve Dev and Kamia's relationship. I never met Kamia, much less asked what helped her repair things with her mom. But if the research above is any indication, trust, safety, and an increased willingness to engage, even when it was unpleasant to do so, probably had something to do with it.

CLAIM #2: VALIDATION WILL HELP YOU MANAGE CONFLICT

Researchers Laurence and Emily Alison from the University of Liverpool disproved the popular notion that torture is an effective method of obtaining credible information from detainees during interrogations (situations defined by conflict). Their extensive research shows that torture actually impairs communication and recall, increases resistance, damages the reliability of any information obtained, and culminates in disengagement, withdrawal, and psychological trauma.[6] What is effective? Rapport-oriented approaches, such as the one they developed based on modern psychotherapy. Rapport is more or less synonymous with validation and includes techniques such as "finding common ground, engaging in self-disclosure, and displaying understanding via empathy."[7] Studies have conclusively shown that rapport strategies are more likely to secure information and decrease tactical resistance from detainees, while accusatorial approaches—sarcasm, intimidation, appearing judgmental, etc.—have the opposite effect.[8]

If you've ever been in a "conversation" with a customer service representative that felt more like a terrorist interrogation, you probably won't be surprised to learn that validation has proven critical to staving off conflict and ensuring constructive communication in this domain as well. Validation has been shown to decrease defensiveness and sustain positive customer relations, resulting in customers who are more satisfied with how their problem is resolved. Conversely, when service representatives do not apologize or fail to really "hear" the customer's concerns, the conversation is likely to escalate such that the problem becomes unresolvable.[9] (Comcast, I hope you're reading this.) I should note that validation has proven equally effective, and indeed critical, to conflict management in marital and parent-child relationships as well. It features prominently in various approaches that have been shown to improve both types of relationships.

Using validation during conflicts is like adding an adorable cat filter to yourself during a videoconferencing meeting—it makes you immediately less threatening and infinitely harder to argue with. Why? The answer appears to be in how it affects the validated person's physiology. As someone becomes more upset, their ability to reason, recall, and focus sharply decreases. Essentially, the cognitive faculties needed to process information and problem-solve go out the window. Their sympathetic nervous system takes over, and their response options are reduced to fight, flight, or freeze.

Validation tempers this response—it decreases sympathetic

arousal and increases a person's ability to reason and engage in perspective-taking.[10] Validating people in highly stressful situations, such as those posed by conflicts, has been shown to decrease their heart rate, galvanic skin response (sweating), and negative emotions.[11] Not surprisingly, invalidation has proven to have the opposite effect—it increases physiological arousal, limiting one's ability to respond rationally, resulting in conflict escalation.[12]

CLAIM #3: VALIDATING PEOPLE WILL INCREASE YOUR INFLUENCE

For our purposes, the term *influencing people* means getting them to listen to you. You give advice; they take it. You tell them what to do; they do it. Note that your influence won't extend very far if people aren't engaging with you. As a doctor, Dev had all sorts of great advice and resources for her daughter, but Kamia wouldn't speak to her. If you want to increase your influence, you need to get people to listen to *and* talk to you. Validation is a bit of a silver bullet in this regard, as it has proven to do both.

Getting People to Talk

As I mentioned, people are more likely to trust someone who validates them. Interestingly, trust is its own sort of truth serum—it gets people talking. Research on intimate and sibling relationships confirms that people are more likely to open up to those they trust, while findings from workplace settings reveal that people prioritize trustworthiness over warmth and expertise in deciding who they'll discuss their problems with.[13] These outcomes are consistent with research by Christina Gamache Martin and colleagues at the University of Oregon, who studied adolescents' behavior when sharing an emotionally upsetting experience with their mothers for the first time.[14] Gamache Martin's research showed that when teens don't expect their moms to be validating, they end up talking less and keeping the most meaningful parts of the experience to themselves. In other words, the less validated and accepted a teen expects to be, the more likely they are to give a G-rated trailer version of their experience; only moms who can be counted on for validation get to see what's really going on.

Validation's effects on self-disclosure hold true even for strangers.[15] Upon meeting for the first time, people who are validated during an initial conversation share more personal details and report increased feelings of social connection compared to those who have pleasant conversations that lack validation. **Taken as a whole, the research is clear: validation is a surefire way to get people talking.**

Getting People to Listen

Importantly, validation inclines people not only to talk but also to listen. There's *a lot* of research in this space, but the most compelling comes from studies on the most notoriously stubborn, unpersuadable, cannot-be-reasoned-with people on the planet—adolescents. A study at Columbia University of more than five hundred mothers and adolescents found that teens who said their mothers consistently use just one validation skill—self-disclosure*—viewed their moms as being more trustworthy and having more expertise compared to teens whose mothers rarely or never use this skill.[16] This, in turn, predicted teens' intentions to smoke cigarettes and have sexual intercourse. You read that correctly: when asked if they intended to smoke or have sex, teens who reported that their mothers frequently used this one validation skill were more likely to say no.**

In an even more shocking study published in the *Journal of Interpersonal Violence*, researchers looked at the relationship between adolescent adversity, validation, and dating violence.[17] They found that adolescents who were exposed to recent hardships, like

---

* Note: Disclosure is a validation skill. This can be confusing, given that it also compels others to talk, or self-disclose, more.
** Fun fact: Research suggests that behavioral intentions reliably predict future behavior. (Thomas L. Webb and Paschal Sheeran, "Does Changing Behavioral Intentions Engender Behavior Change? A Meta-Analysis of the Experimental Evidence," *Psychological Bulletin* 132, no. 2 [January 1, 2006]: 249–68, https://doi.org/10.1037/0033-2909.132.2.249.)

receiving a poor report card, having parents who recently divorced, or lacking close friends, were more likely to become perpetrators and/or victims of dating violence. But the connection between hardships and dating violence was found only in teens who perceived their mothers as providing low or average levels of validation. When mothers' validation was high, the relationship between hardships and dating violence disappeared. High rates of validation from fathers had a similar effect on the relationship between hardship and *perpetration* of violence, but only in *boys*. I feel like this study warrants a public service announcement: **Parents, if your adolescents are struggling, validating them may protect them from becoming victims or perpetrators of sexual violence.**

We can presume the parents in these studies did not want their kids to smoke, have sex, or engage in sexual violence, yet they didn't necessarily say so. It wasn't finger-wagging that proved effective in these studies; it was the soft touch of validation that ultimately influenced kids' intentions and behavior.

CLAIM #4: VALIDATION DRIVES BIG CHANGES

It obviously feels good to be validated. The question is, how good? Good enough to, say, get your kid to clean the garage while you work out on the elliptical watching old seasons of *Survivor*? At this point, I had hoped to present exhibit A—a picture of me getting my workout on while my daughter, Havana, picked up the garage floor, but my editor said it was too grainy, so you'll have to take my word that it happened.

The question of whether or not validation feels good enough to entice a kid to clean the garage is an empirical one. We must determine if it's sufficiently *rewarding*. **Anything that's rewarding has the potential to act as "positive reinforcement"—a reward given *after* a behavior that increases the likelihood that the behavior will be repeated.** If validating Havana after she cleans the garage while I'm working out motivates her to start cleaning the garage the next time I hop on the elliptical, I know my validation worked to positively reinforce her behavior.

In the studies on influence I discussed earlier, validation always came before the behavior in question: people were validated *before* smoking, and high rates of parental validation appeared to *protect* adolescents from dating violence. When validation has an effect on a behavior before it occurs, we can say it influenced that behavior. This is different from what happens when validation reinforces a behavior after the fact. Positive reinforcements have a much more powerful effect on behavior and can drive people to endure all sorts of conditions in the hopes of getting the "payout" they seek (e.g., consider the Herculean effort Olympic athletes put into training in the hopes of bringing home a gold medal).

Positive reinforcements operate by lighting up the reward center of our brain and causing the release of neurotransmitters like dopamine that cause us to feel pleasure. Opioids, orgasms, and cash giveaways, for example, all have this effect. Neuroimaging research has shown that feeling understood activates these same reward centers of the brain and also regions associated with social connectedness.[18] Going back to our original question of whether validation feels good enough to cause people to change their behavior, the answer is a resounding yes.

The unprecedented power that comes from communicating acceptance can change a great many things, including what a person will do in the future. The details around how to use validation like I did with Havana to drive very specific changes are covered in part 3, where I'll explain some of the change strategies I used in addition to positive reinforcement to transform cleaning the garage into a game my daughter wanted to play.

For now, I'll conclude with two important points. First, you should never underestimate the power of verbal rewards like validation and positive feedback. Compared to tangible reinforcements like prizes and money, which have been shown to *decrease* a person's internal motivation over time, verbal rewards have proven to *increase* it.[19] Second, validation cannot be faked. (Comcast, I hope you're listening.) It's thus well suited for reinforcing behaviors that benefit the person we're reinforcing or are mutually beneficial. I genuinely believe, for instance, that it's important for Havana to help out and take pride in contributing to the family. One could arguably feign mindfulness, understanding, and empathy, but that is neither what this book nor validation are about.

CLAIM #5: VALIDATION FOSTERS SELF-COMPASSION

As I write this, I'm distracted by pangs of shame and the thought: "I'm a bad parent." I know, *exactly* what you want to hear from the person who claims she can help you transform your life and relationships. Sitting on the floor next to me, Havana is crestfallen, having just been told that I need some quiet time before we can play another game of "blindfolded chess." No, she's not a prodigy; she makes me wear the blindfold so that I clumsily knock over all the pieces every time I make a move. In my defense, we've played six games in a row and I'm behind on my emails, which I'm also clearly avoiding in favor of writing. In her defense, she's sick with COVID-19. (Note: this was still in the pre-Omicron days, before vaccinations were available to children, and relatively few people had been diagnosed with COVID.)

Despite all the sheltering, we failed to keep her safe, and now I'm too busy to play with her. Full disclosure: I don't want to play with her. I'm out of steam. Between the terror of seeing her struggle to breathe at night, the exhaustion of being her emotional punching bag this week, and trying to conduct telehealth sessions from my closet with suicidal clients, I'm utterly depleted. I've decided to distract myself with work rather than play another game with my sad, sick child. I now realize my "invalidation radar" has been tripped. I'm detecting invalidation somewhere in my environment. Reader, it appears to be coming from inside the house! Time to call in the self-validation troops!

Self-validation simply means applying to yourself the skills you use to validate others. You can think of it as an exercise in self-compassion. In *The Mindful Self-Compassion Workbook*, leading experts Kristin Neff and Christopher Germer describe self-compassion as "treating yourself the way you would treat a friend who is having a hard time—even if your friend blew it or is feeling inadequate. . ."[20] The ability to validate yourself is a facet of self-compassion.

None of us actively choose to berate or invalidate ourselves. These are learned behaviors. Internalized messages. The degree to which we internalize invalidation from others becomes abundantly clear when you look at research on mental health disorders. Symptoms of depression, anxiety, borderline personality disorder, post-traumatic stress disorder (PTSD), narcissism, and even psychopathy are all many times higher in those exposed to pervasive invalidation—families or environments that consistently and routinely dismiss, punish, and challenge a person's expressed thoughts and emotions.[21] **As I see it, the current "mental health crisis" is in part a "validation crisis."** That is not to say that everyone who grew up or lives in an invalidating environment will develop mental health problems, or that people struggling with them have necessarily been exposed to pervasive invalidation. The point is that people who are frequently and consistently invalidated by others are *more likely* to experience mental health problems characterized by self-invalidation and self-loathing.

Sadly, invalidation doesn't just occur in families; it echoes throughout our culture. A 2021 study published by the American Psychological Association showed that multiracial individuals experience various types of *racial identity invalidation*—having inaccurate racial categorization imposed upon them by others—and that it contributes to negative health effects **above and beyond** those resulting from other forms of discrimination.[22] Identity invalidation has been reported in upward of 85 percent of bisexuals, while nonbinary adolescents report pervasive invalidation across various social contexts contributing to internalized shame, self-doubt, and mental health problems and correlating with high rates of self-harm and suicide attempts.[23]

Finally, pervasive invalidation has proven to be a unique contributor to gender inequality, while the denial, minimization, and silencing of women's perspectives are theorized to play a causal role in gender-based violence against women.[24] The investigations into Jeffrey Epstein and R. Kelly are two devastating high-profile examples of how pervasive invalidation contributes to violence against women.

Fortunately, just as self-invalidation is a learned behavior, self-validation also can be learned. One of the main reasons therapists are trained to validate their clients is to show them how to validate themselves. Sure, validation is a great way for a therapist to improve the therapeutic relationship, manage conflict, influence behavior, and reinforce progress. But often the biggest change people need to make is in how they relate to themselves. My job is to validate the valid thoughts and emotions my clients have been taught to dismiss so that they can learn to do the same for themselves.

The relationship we have with ourselves is like any other. The skills you use to cultivate and communicate acceptance to others are no less effective when you direct them inward to temper your own self-judgments, as I'll explain in chapter 18. **The paradox that those skilled in validating come to appreciate is that not only do we need to treat others the way we'd want to be treated, but we also must treat ourselves with the same kindness we'd extend to others.** In case you're wondering, I've decided that my desire for rest and distraction is valid and that I should hold off on another round of blindfolded chess. At least for now.

CONCLUSION

It's one thing to say that validation skills can help you improve your relationships, decrease conflict, influence people, drive change, and develop self-compassion; it's another to say that *anyone* can develop these skills. The question of whether or not you need to be emotionally intelligent or have an advanced degree in psychology to become good at validating can be answered through experimental research. And it has been. From family members[25] to students[26] and doctors,[27] people from all walks of life have proven capable of increasing the extent to which others perceive them as validating *and* achieving positive outcomes like those discussed in this chapter. Significant changes have been reported after just two sessions[28] of validation training, and in one experiment after only forty-five minutes.[29] These studies show not only that everyday folks are able to objectively increase their ability to validate through basic instruction, but also that they can achieve meaningful improvements in their lives and relationships as a result.

In my experience, one of the greatest predictors of a person's success with validation is the degree to which they understand the concept. Is it possible to validate someone who's being irrational? What if you don't understand or empathize with the other person's position? To navigate these and other issues that arise while practicing validation, you'll need more than a surface definition of the term. Having established how relationship saving, conflict mediating, change facilitating, and self-affirming validation is, we now turn to what it means to actually validate someone.

CHAPTER 3

WHAT IT MEANS TO BE SEEN— VALIDATION DEFINED

I like good strong words that mean something.

—LOUISA MAY ALCOTT, *LITTLE WOMEN*

I'm going to let you in on a secret. It's not a secret, really, so much as a question. Early in my training, I was told to ask myself this question anytime a client came to me with a problem. I saw no reason why I should be this thoughtful only with my clients, and I have tried to keep this question in mind whenever *anyone* comes to me for support, including myself.* I can honestly say that doing so has made me an infinitely more effective therapist, mother, daughter, consultant, sister, spouse, friend, and colleague. The question is simple: **"Should I respond with problem-solving or validation?"**

This question is intended to challenge one of our more endearing characteristics: we want to make things better. When someone is upset or comes to us with a problem, we want to take away their pain and help them find a solution. Unfortunately, as well intentioned as we may be, our efforts often backfire. Rather than solving problems, we make them worse. Instead of reassuring people, we invalidate their distress.

Consider an example as old as time: shortly after a family

---

* Yes, I come to myself for support on the regular. It's one of the perks of being a good psychologist. Just kidding. It's a perk of being able to self-validate, which I'll show you how to do in chapter 18.

welcomes home their new baby girl, the now "big brother" declares that he hates her. "No, you love your sister," the parents reassure him. "She's just a baby now, but you'll be playing together in no time!" Of course, that baby isn't going to be a suitable playmate for a couple of years. Which in kid time is, like, forever! Either the little boy will quietly remain confused and hurt by his parents' reaction, or he'll escalate and possibly end up punished for an outburst. Far from "cheered up," most kids in this scenario will feel invalidated.

If you can relate to the parents in this example, or recall instances when you did something similar, don't worry, so can I! My instincts are constantly overriding my thought process, especially when it comes to my kid, whose problems I feel biologically driven to solve. Pain? I will absorb it! Doubt? I will relieve it! Are those tears I see? I'll contort my face and make fart sounds till she starts laughing. Our innate drive to find solutions is fine in some scenarios, just not *all* scenarios. The problem with problem-solving is that oftentimes when people come to us with an issue, they're not looking for us to resolve it; they're seeking validation.

Responding initially with validation does not preclude you from following up later with problem-solving or vice versa. For instance, you might immediately validate your partner's distress after they botched a job interview and then later explore what they might do differently next time. **You can and should toggle between validation and problem-solving, responding with what you think is needed in the moment. But at any given time, assume you can offer only one or the other.**

The definition of problem-solving is straightforward—it's the process of finding solutions to problems. I'll talk more about problem-solving and other "change strategies" in part 3. For now, though, I'm going to focus on validation so that you're crystal clear on what it is and what it isn't. For this chapter, I encourage you to table any fantasies you might be entertaining about the people you hope to change and instead focus on wrapping your head around this concept. Consider this a test of your validation potential and first lesson: **One's ability to flexibly move between focusing on change and validation determines how successful they will be in either pursuit.**

WHAT'S IN A WORD?

I earlier defined validation as communication that one is *mindful*, *understands*, and *empathizes* with another person's *experience*, thereby accepting it as *valid*. The first part of that definition is about how to validate someone—you need to demonstrate mindfulness, understanding, and empathy. So what, exactly, does that mean?

Mindfulness

Mindfulness, you might remember, is defined by Jon Kabat-Zinn as "paying attention, on purpose, in the present moment and non-judgmentally." With validation, you bring that purposeful, nonjudgmental awareness to another person. In a sense, validation is a kind of *interpersonal mindfulness practice*—rather than the breath or body serving as the anchor for your attention, as is common in traditional mindfulness exercises, your focus is on another person's experience.

Various issues can compromise our ability to be mindful of others, but two are worth highlighting because they are among the most common and least obvious. The first is that we tend to *overestimate* the extent to which we're paying attention, particularly when we're convinced that we understand or care about something. Television shows like *Undercover Boss*, which use the premise of having a boss pretend to be a new employee within the company they manage, highlight this issue. The boss always appears to have a sophisticated understanding of how the company operates before going undercover. Without fail, after spending a week in the trenches observing their employees, the boss develops greater gratitude for them and insight into what it actually takes to run the company. Yes, they're contrived, but these shows nonetheless illustrate a very real phenomena—observing and being mindful of people's experiences allow us to connect with them in ways we otherwise couldn't. They also highlight that working toward a shared goal or orbiting around someone is different from truly paying attention to them.

Ironically, the second issue that can compromise our ability to be mindful of others is self-awareness. When we know that we don't understand or emotionally connect with another person's experience, we tend to recoil. We're quick to assume that our ignorance or lack of immediate interest will cause us to say or do something offensive, so we end up doing nothing at all. Not even listening. We change topics, look at our phones, or otherwise disengage. But the truth is, you don't need to deeply understand or empathize with another person's experience to bear witness to it. Indeed, it is hard to arrive at understanding or empathy if you haven't been paying attention.

Understanding

In terms of validation, understanding means seeing a person's reaction, or some part of it, as logical or justifiable. Unfortunately, rather than attending to the aspects of someone's response that are reasonable, we tend to focus on what's "wrong." You can thank the negativity bias for that.[1]

The negativity bias is like a little shoulder devil whose sole mission in life is to draw our attention toward what's wrong, bad, or threatening in our environment. Evolutionarily speaking, this biased little devil has served us well: we're more likely to survive if our attention is drawn to a lion's bared teeth, rather than his beautiful, Mufasa-esque mane. Interpersonally, though, the negativity bias can be problematic. To validate someone, you must ignore what's wrong with their perspective—however obvious it may be— and instead focus on what's valid. The key to thriving and not just surviving in your relationships is to ignore the fangs and focus first on the mane.

Empathy

Empathy means to connect with another person's emotions. In the context of validation, it also can mean to attach meaning to someone's experience or to demonstrate care. Empathy here is based on logical reasoning and is born out of understanding. I was able to empathize with the embarrassment my friend felt after her adult son walked in on her and her husband having sex not only because I know what embarrassment feels like, but also because her reaction made logical sense.

Empathy often gets confused with sympathy, which is understandable. I mean, we shouldn't be expected to differentiate words that literally and figuratively rhyme! It doesn't really matter if you confuse these concepts in conversation or when purchasing Hallmark cards, but for the purposes of validation, the differences between them are important: sympathy is a reaction to another person's suffering or negative circumstances; empathy is about connecting with another person's emotions, be they good or bad. Whereas sympathy means feeling bad *for* someone, empathy is feeling *with* them; sympathy looks down from on high and says, "That sucks"; empathy comes down to eye level and says, "I feel you."

In the summer of 2021, my mother was diagnosed with a brain tumor and required emergency surgery to remove it. Thankfully, the surgery was a resounding success and she's since made a full recovery. During this time, I was working with a client, Ella, who lost her mom to cancer at a young age. Once I'd had a glimpse of what it might be like to lose my own mother, I was overcome with empathy for Ella. In the weeks when things were touch and go with my mom, the fear and sorrow were overwhelming at times; I couldn't imagine how I would have managed the situation if I had been only a child.

After my mom had recovered, I chose to share my experience with Ella in an effort to validate some of the emotions she had around her loss.* During the discussion, I felt the familiar connection that only validation affords. Later that day, I received an email from Ella. It was only a few sentences long, but in that space, she managed to validate *my* experience like no one else had. I wasn't seeking her validation; I didn't expect or pull for it, but I'd be lying if I said I wasn't moved by her words. Ella wasn't overcome by a need to take care of me. My vulnerability didn't spin her out the way some might assume it would. I'd seen myself in her, which simply allowed her to see herself in me. Empathy often has this effect; sympathy does not.

Note that experiencing empathy and conveying it are two different things. If Ella and I hadn't communicated our empathy, neither one of us would have felt validated by the other. Moreover, if we'd been ineffective in our communication, we wouldn't have felt validated, either. This is a subtle but critical point. I mentioned earlier that emotionally sensitive people are often less inclined to practice validation skills because they can easily connect with others' emotions. They make the mistake of assuming that their unique ability to empathize means they are equally effective at *communicating* their empathy. But that's not necessarily the case.

Sensitive people are often subjected to a dizzying combination of too much and too little feedback regarding their feelings, which can make learning how to communicate them challenging. A person who quickly detects and experiences emotions deeply is also more prone to getting overwhelmed by them. Even if the individual manages to keep from getting dysregulated, their reactions are often bigger than those around them. After years of being directly or indirectly punished for being "so emotional," many sensitive people learn to repress rather than express negative feelings. On the other hand, when they do communicate more "appropriate" emotions like care or empathy, they rarely get the feedback

---

* I'll describe how to safely use Disclosure to validate someone in chapter 13.

required to help them consistently stick the landing. Few people are going to tell someone who is attempting to empathize with them that they're coming on too strong or missing the mark. **Having learned that they connect all too easily with people's emotions, but not realizing that their empathy doesn't necessarily translate, many with the power of sensitivity overlook the utility of learning how to communicate it effectively.**

A Word About Authenticity

Wrapping up this discussion on the components of validation, I want to highlight that you should think of validation as a matter of degrees: the degree to which you communicate it depends on the amount of mindfulness, understanding, and empathy you can authentically convey. Inauthentic validation is not validation at all. It's manipulation, exploitation, or possibly ignorance, but it's not validation. As crafty as you might be, trust me when I say that you should not fake validation in the hope of achieving the positive transformations it promises. It won't work. Inauthenticity comes at a cost, and that cost includes the very mindfulness, understanding, and empathy that are required to transform others without compromising your relationships with them.

WHAT TO VALIDATE

Validation communicates that you're mindful (paying attention), understand (see rationality in), and empathize with (connect with or care about) someone's *experience*, thereby accepting it as *valid*. So what constitutes a person's experience, and how do you know if it's valid?

For our purposes, a person's experience consists of their *emotions, thoughts,* and *behavior*. Importantly, you do not need to validate each part of someone's experience. One of the cardinal rules of validation is that you should only validate the valid. Remember, the negativity bias causes us to focus on what we dislike or find confusing. Your task is to search for the "kernel of truth"—what you consider reasonable—in another person's experience, and validate it. If you're struggling to find the kernel of truth, consider whether their emotions, behavior, or thoughts make

ONLY VALIDATE THE VALID.

sense in light of each other. Does a person's behavior seem valid given their thoughts? Organizing a demonstration to demand that the government provide nuclear waste cleanup is reasonable if someone thinks their city has been exposed to radioactive particles. Are their emotions reasonable given their behavior? Feeling paranoid about a potential alien invasion is understandable if a person hasn't slept in three days and has been binge-watching alien documentaries.

Just as you should demonstrate mindfulness, understanding, and empathy only to the extent that you can do so authentically, you also should validate a person's thoughts, behaviors, or emotions only if you legitimately consider them to be valid. Again, only validate the valid.

The *in*valid reactions are what you might work to change. I was once treating a patient with schizophrenia who abruptly went off his meds and became convinced that I was colluding with the government to have him killed. I did not see any validity in his thoughts because I was obviously not in cahoots with the federal government. The emotions of fear and distrust he expressed seemed reasonable to me, as did his efforts to contact a lawyer, seeing as how he thought I was plotting to kill him. I wasn't going to get anywhere by openly challenging his thoughts. Instead, I needed to focus on validating his emotions and behavior and then work backward from there.

You may not frequently find yourself in the position of having to validate someone with schizophrenia, but in a world as divided as ours, you can probably relate to the challenge of trying to find the kernel of truth in another person's response when so much of it seems senseless or even dangerous. These are the times when validation is most important.

This emphasis on "only validating the valid" raises an important question: how do you know if someone's thoughts, behaviors, or emotions are valid?

Thoughts are considered valid when they are logical, based on facts, and grounded in reality. People are constantly making assumptions and interpretations based on the facts of a situation, and they inevitably arrive at different conclusions. As long as someone's deductions are logical or plausible, you can consider them valid. Note: you don't need to *agree* with another person's perspective for it to be logical. More on this later.

Valid behaviors are those that are appropriate in terms of cultural norms or *effective* with respect to the individual's goals and the context (past or present).* The "culturally appropriate" criteria can be problematic because cultural norms may conflict with a person's values or be oppressive and worth challenging. Rosa Parks, for instance, violated cultural norms by refusing to sit in the back of the bus. Her behavior was consistent with her values and a remarkably effective form of social protest, despite the fact that she was bucking cultural norms. Because cultural norms can be thorny, I tend to focus more on whether a person's behavior is *effective* given their long-term goals and the situation. For example, if you find out that your partner has been cheating on you for the last eight months, feelings of betrayal, anger, and disbelief are all valid emotions. The thought "I don't ever want to see my partner again" might also be valid. Burning down your partner's house, however, is NOT a valid reaction because it will most definitely create more problems for you than it resolves, and it likely conflicts with some of your goals (unless you value arson and prison time).

A person's behavior may be valid in terms of the past, even if it's not in the present. When I was working as a lab manager in my first job after college, I automatically defaulted to raising my hand in meetings when I had something to say. I worried my immaturity

---

* Behaviors that are driven by normal biological functioning, like going to the bathroom or drinking water, are also considered valid.

might be reflecting poorly on my boss, so I decided to speak with her about it. When I did, she just smiled. "You've been in school your whole life," she said. "Give your brain some time to update." Raising my hand, and sometimes shaking it dramatically to avoid being passed over for the boy next to me, was effective in helping me reach my goals in school. My boss recognized the validity in my behavior, even though it wasn't effective in the moment.

Finally, **emotions are always valid.** Okay, maybe they're not *always* valid, but it's rarely effective to challenge people's emotions, unlike their thoughts and behaviors. I'll discuss the rare situations in which invalidating someone's emotion might be appropriate in chapter 11, but for the most part, telling someone how they should feel, or that their feelings are "wrong," doesn't typically turn out well. At best, you get into an argument neither side can win. At worst, you cause someone to distrust their emotions in ways that can deeply distort how they see themselves and the world. Although there's nothing wrong with trying to change someone's emotions by, say, cheering them up or calming them down, you want to steer clear of invalidating them by suggesting that they shouldn't feel whatever they're feeling. There's a world of difference between helping someone regulate their emotions: "It sucks to feel like people are judging your parenting. Let's try to find something to take your mind off things," and invalidating them: "Why do you care what other people think?"

Technically speaking—but remember, you're not going to invalidate people's emotions, so it doesn't matter—emotions are considered valid when they are proportionate to the situation that provoked them and normative, expected, or understandable given the circumstances. To determine if someone's behavior is "understandable given the circumstances," you need to know the circumstances. But you can only ever know a small fraction of what's going on in another person's life at any given moment. Even if you could follow them around all day, your insights would still be limited to what you can directly observe. Physical pain, brain chemistry, hormone levels—none of this stuff is observable, yet it all has a profound effect on how a person feels and responds to their environment.

If you're really struggling to see the validity in someone's emotions, you can ask questions, get curious, or focus on any invalid behavior, particularly if it's egregious: for example, "Havana, screaming at the top of your lungs is not going to get you what you want." You might help someone identify or label their emotions, but for your sake and theirs, don't invalidate them.

WHAT VALIDATION ISN'T

Most of the obstacles you're likely to run into with validation can be avoided simply by understanding what it is not.

Validation ≠ Agreement

I'm a vegetarian for environmental and ethical reasons. Over the years, I've had hundreds of conversations with people on this issue and have found a lot to validate in the perspectives of meat-eaters. I generally don't agree with or like where they land on this issue, but I can almost always find something to validate.

"I don't cook and don't trust that I could get my nutritional needs met otherwise." *Makes sense. We are all spread stupidly thin, and overhauling your entire diet is pretty daunting.*

"I'm just one person; why does it even matter?" *Fair point. I wonder about this, too, sometimes.*

"If I'm going to stop eating meat, I should stop eating dairy, too, or using any animal-based products. I don't think that would be healthy or sustainable." *Tell me about it! I failed in my efforts to go vegan. I wrestle with the hypocrisy of my lifestyle every day.*

To be clear, I don't agree with these perspectives. I have plenty of "yeah, but" counterpoints, and if I was trying to challenge someone's opinion, I might voice them. But if I'm trying to validate—to show some degree of awareness, understanding, and empathy toward their position and accept where they are—I need to focus only on what's valid. Because I see the logic and rationality in these perspectives, I should communicate that, not the extent to which I disagree.

Note that validating one part of a person's experience (e.g., their emotions) doesn't necessarily reinforce or reward the aspects you want to change (e.g., their behavior). I once worked with a high-powered exec who wanted help with anger management. One day she came to me, wondering how to deal with what we can all agree is the most offensive behavior on the face of the planet—her neighbors had started putting their trash in her receptacle. Each week when garbage night came, my client would lug her trash out to the curb only to find that they had filled up their trash bin *and hers.* I feel my blood starting to boil just thinking about it. She wanted to go over to their place after work and tell them off. Instead, I worked with her to craft an email that was both assertive and gentle. Reader, the message we drafted was a masterpiece. A real work of art. She sent it to them and forwarded their response to me a few hours later. It did the trick! They apologized, expressed remorse, and even invited her over for a game night. All was right in the world.

Three weeks later, I awoke in the middle of the night to a call from the police department. It was my client. Apparently, her neighbors had once again put their trash in her bin. Feeling enraged and defeated, she decided to get even by slashing the tires of their new car. In a shared parking garage. Where there was video surveillance. When the police arrived to question her, she resisted arrest and was taken into custody. As she relayed these details to me, she ping-ponged between defensiveness and guilt. I stayed quiet and let her talk. The first thought that went through my mind/ entire body was, "How could she do that?!" The first thing I said was, "Seeing their garbage in your bin must have felt like a slap in the face." I meant it. She'd worked so hard to be effective, had success, lost that success, and in the end had nothing to show for it other than a sense of disrespect and a bag of her own trash. It wasn't my *first* reaction to her story. But it wasn't far behind.

To my surprise, she broke down crying. I spent the next ten minutes just listening and validating her thoughts and emotions. This in no way suggested that I thought she'd managed them effectively (i.e., that her behavior was valid). On the contrary, validating how she felt set the stage for me to ultimately compel her to take responsibility for her behavior, repair things with her neighbors, and commit to working on tolerating strong emotions without acting on them. Had I come down hard on what she'd done, I'd have stood little chance of influencing what she did next. **People are far more likely to listen to what you have to say about their behavior if they trust that you accept and understand the reasoning or emotions behind it.**

Validation ≠ Praise or Approval

As I mentioned in chapter 1, validation is often confused with praise or approval. This is why people say it's bad to rely on "external validation." Their point is that trying to photoshop or change yourself to impress others will only make it harder for you to accept yourself as you are. And that's true. Contorting yourself to earn people's approval will absolutely hurt your sense of self-worth, not help it. An identity that's built on facades is like a house made out of paper—it won't hold up. But validation communicates acceptance, not judgment. It doesn't pat the head; it touches the heart. Someone who adds a bulging-eye emoji to a selfie you posted is saying, "I like the way you look." This is a judgment, albeit a positive one, and a compliment. Validation is neither of these things. Validation says, "I accept who you are, regardless of how you look." People struggling with low self-esteem and insecurity need more validation, not less. They need to feel accepted for who they are, independent of how they look or perform.

Validation ≠ Problem-Solving

And now we've come full circle! As I stated at the beginning of this chapter, validation is kind of the opposite of problem-solving: whereas validation communicates acceptance of things as they are, problem-solving communicates an eagerness to change them. When Havana comes home from school crying because she got a bad grade on her spelling test and I respond by brainstorming what she could do differently next time to better prepare, I'm problem-solving her behavior, or helping her determine what she can *change* to get a better outcome in the future. When I say, "Think about how well you've done on all your other spelling tests," I'm problem-solving her thoughts—I'm trying to help her generate alternative ways of thinking about the situation to *change* her perspective. Problem-solving her behavior and thoughts are both indirect attempts to intervene on her emotions or *change* how she feels.

If instead I put my arm around her and say, "Oh, I'm sorry, babe. You must be so disappointed," I'm directly validating her emotions—it's valid to be disappointed after not doing well on something you care about. If I say, "I remember going into the bathroom to cry once after failing a quiz," I'm validating her behavior—it's reasonable to cry when you are upset or disappointed. You could argue that I'm validating her only in an effort to change how she feels, which is true on some level. This book's whole premise is that validation fosters change. The distinction is that when I'm validating someone, I'm not focused on a specific outcome. Again, validation is like a mindfulness exercise in which the object of your focus is another person's experience. In my example, I'm not looking at the clock, wondering how long it's going to take for Havana to compose herself, or thinking through study strategies I might help her develop once I've convinced her that I get it. I'm sitting with the fact that things are as they "should" be in any given moment. Whatever a person's reaction is, it's grounded in a long chain of cause and effect. **Validation communicates that "It's okay." Not, "It will be okay." Affirming the former can position you as an ally; if you**

jump too quickly to the latter, you might very well become part of the problem.

Although validation and problem-solving represent opposite motivations, they're not incompatible. Remember, acceptance and change are like two sides of the same coin. Problem-solving how my kid can better prepare for tests in the future is totally reasonable and may even be necessary if she's struggling to improve her scores. The issue is that in the absence of validation, she's not likely to listen to any of my brilliant ideas. If someone responds to your vulnerability by telling you all of the changes you need to make to feel less vulnerable, you're more likely to feel judged than supported. **Feeling judged translates to feeling misunderstood, and when we don't feel like someone understands us or our problems, we're not likely to trust their advice on how to change things.**

The question of whether the situation warrants validation or problem-solving applies to you as well. Knowing what you need from someone will make you more likely to actually receive it. Remember, problem-solving stems from people's desire to help. If you can tell others where to direct their efforts—"I need to be heard," "I want to feel like someone else understands this," or "I need to know I'm not crazy," for example—they're more likely to hit the target.

RECAP

Validation communicates that you are mindful (nonjudgmentally aware), understand (see rationality in), and empathize with (connect with or care about) someone's experience (emotions, thoughts, or behaviors), thereby accepting it as valid (justifiable, effective, logical). In addition to this comprehensive definition, I want to underscore the points that I find myself repeating most often to my clients and students. Getting the following list tattooed on your forearm would basically be like cheating at validation because you'd have the answers to two-thirds of the problems you're likely to run into up your sleeve.

Points to Remember/Fierce Forearm Tattoos

- Only validate the valid.
- Communicate validation only to the degree that you can do so authentically.
- Validation ≠ agreement.
- Validation ≠ praise or approval.
- Validation ≠ problem-solving.

VALIDATION AND THE ART OF SUFFERING—ONE LAST REASON TO DROP EVERYTHING AND LEARN TO VALIDATE

If there is a meaning in life at all, then there must be meaning in suffering. Suffering is an ineradicable part of life, even as fate and death. Without suffering and death human life cannot be complete.

—VIKTOR FRANKL, *MAN'S SEARCH FOR MEANING*

"I have multiple sclerosis," I said with tears in my eyes.

Marsha Linehan stared at me blankly. "So what?" she asked.

This, reader, was not the response I was expecting from the person who'd revolutionized modern psychology with her insights on validation.

"So, I can't be a DBT therapist."

"Wait, what?" she asked, scrunching her nose.

It was 2011, and I'd spent the last five years in a doctoral program at Duke University learning everything I could about borderline personality disorder (BPD). Pervasive invalidation is believed to play a causal role in BPD, a disorder defined by impulsivity, self-harm, intense mood swings, and anger. Clients with this condition are highly stigmatized within the mental health community and often discriminated against by providers.* From the moment I learned about BPD, I determined that it wasn't enough to not be part of the problem; I needed to be part of the solution. After I completed my doctorate, I was selected for a fellowship in Dialectical Behavior Therapy (DBT)—the first proven treatment for BPD—at a prestigious practice in Seattle, Washington. Within weeks of starting, the other fellows and I were invited to go on a training retreat with Marsha Linehan, the creator of the treatment I'd set out to master. I was at the top of my game, finally in a position to launch a career that would enable me to work with the clients I desperately wanted to serve. Unfortunately, it was looking like I'd have to retire before I'd even begun.

Let me back up. During the second year of my doctoral program, I developed chronic nausea. I'd go to bed wanting to puke. I'd wake up wanting to puke. Years of medical tests offered no answers. Over time, other strange symptoms cropped up, and at the end of my last semester at Duke, I was referred to a neurologist. By that point, I was preparing to move cross-country for an internship in Seattle. The neurologist suggested we run some tests to rule out a neurological explanation for my symptoms. He said he was confident they'd be negative. Famous last words.

---

* It is not uncommon for therapists to refuse to work with people who suffer from BPD or to refer them out at the first sign of trouble (aka BPD symptoms). As one eminent psychologist once told me, "I don't work with 'borderlines' because I don't like being sued, lied to, and threatened." That was putting it mildly. *Crazy, insane, two-faced, a real piece of work,* and *bitch* are all terms I've heard licensed medical professionals use to describe these clients. But here's the thing about BPD: it's three times more likely to occur in women than in men. And not just any women, but those with histories of childhood abuse and sexual trauma. The judgment and bias my field has perpetuated toward those with BPD bring me great shame. It is victim-blaming at its worst. (Paola Bozzatello et al., "The Role of Trauma in Early Onset Borderline Personality Disorder: A Biopsychosocial Perspective," *Frontiers in Psychiatry* 12 [January 1, 2021], https://doi.org/10.3389/fpsyt.2021.721361; Lais Barros De Aquino Ferreira et al., "Borderline Personality Disorder and Sexual Abuse: A Systematic Review," *Psychiatry Research-Neuroimaging* 262 [April 1, 2018]: 70–77, https://doi.org/10.1016/j.psychres.2018.01.043; Jeffrey S. Ball and Paul S. Links, "Borderline Personality Disorder and Childhood Trauma: Evidence for a Causal Relationship," *Current Psychiatry Reports* 11, no. 1 [January 22, 2009]: 63–68, https://doi.org/10.1007/s11920-009-0010-4; Andrew E. Skodol and Donna S. Bender, "Why Are Women Diagnosed Borderline More Than Men?," *Psychiatric Quarterly* 74, no. 4 [January 1, 2003]: 349–60, https://doi.org/10.1023/a:1026087410516.)

Halfway through the road trip west with my now-husband, Mat, the neurologist called. He told me I needed to see a doctor as soon as I arrived in Seattle. "You have MS," he said.

"Like Stephen Hawking?" I asked.

"No. That's ALS."

I clearly had no idea what I was dealing with.

The doctors in Washington confirmed the multiple sclerosis (MS) diagnosis. I spent the next year working and studying during the day while administering shots into my abdomen at night to slow the disease's progression. I experienced fatigue that was unlike anything I'd ever felt before. I would crash on Friday evenings and sleep straight through Sunday, waking only to eat or use the bathroom. At work, I'd lock the door in between patients and curl up under my desk to surf the ebb and flow of nausea as I slipped in and out of sleep.

I was no longer suffering from depression, but after a decade of crafting facades of functioning to mask my mental health symptoms, I'd become pretty adept at channeling pain into productivity and hiding in plain sight. People were always shocked to learn I had MS: "But you seem so healthy!" This was important to me then, and in many ways still is. Be it depression or MS, I've never wanted to give a disease anything it hadn't already taken from me.

I completed the internship, received my PhD, and got married all within a year of the diagnosis. On paper and social media, I was living my best life. Unfortunately, as I transitioned into the DBT fellowship, I was feeling less like I was fighting a disease and more like I was fighting myself.

The position was both a dream come true and a nightmare for someone in my condition. I was practicing alongside some of the best clinicians I'd ever met, doing work that felt deeply important; I was also seeing more clients than I had ever seen, and every single one of them was suicidal, violent, self-harming, or some devastating combination of the three. I was on-call 24/7. My symptoms were flaring, and the seams were starting to show. At one point I threw up in a session. "One moment," I said to the woman who'd just tearfully admitted to cheating on her partner. Knowing I couldn't make it to the bathroom in time, I grabbed the wastepaper basket next to my desk and, as quietly as possible, vomited into it. For the record, I imagine vomiting is the *worst* way a therapist could respond to someone who just confessed to having an affair with her brother in-law.

I realized I was way over the line of perseverance and fortitude. I was in denial. It broke my heart, but I had to accept that, despite how much I loved the work, I wasn't cut out for it. By the time the retreat with Linehan rolled around, I'd decided that my first meeting with her would be my last.

Back to that encounter:

"You're saying you can't be a DBT therapist because you have MS," Linehan stated plainly.

"That's right."

"That's wrong." Perhaps the most *in*validating thing she could have said to me.

"You must be a DBT therapist *because* you have MS," she explained with what sounded like exasperation.

I'd heard Linehan could be sharp, but this was ridiculous. She didn't know anything about me or what I was going through. The mother of validation seemed more concerned with changing a decision that had taken me months to arrive at than accepting me for who I am.

"If you don't like the work, or the patients, or the therapy itself, then you should quit. That's a fact."

"I love all of those things," I told her.

She eyed me skeptically and then asked why DBT appealed to me.

"I think your work on validation was groundbreaking," I said. "It's made me a better person."

"I stole that from Carl Rogers," she said flatly. *

---

* My editor asked me to clarify that Linehan wasn't admitting to actually stealing Carl Rogers's work. She is known for her irreverent sense of humor, which is peppered throughout our conversation and reflected in her comment. I, however, am less

"Really?"

"Sort of," she replied. "But that's exactly why you should be a DBT therapist."

"Carl Rogers?" I asked, confused.

"Validation. Your suffering is a gift. Don't squander it."

Every evening during the retreat, Linehan recited a prayer for all of the people battling mental illness. The ones who felt alone in the world and with their despair. It sounds corny, but the prayer was really quite moving. You could sense her connection to the lives she'd devoted herself to saving. In 2020, just prior to retiring, Linehan published her memoir, *Building a Life Worth Living*. In it, she detailed the emotional suffering she experienced after being institutionalized for several years as a young woman. The symptoms she developed while in the hospital are consistent with BPD, as was the discrimination and mistreatment she received. It's almost impossible to imagine how the young woman she describes, prone to episodes of severe self-harm and suicide attempts, survived, much less succeeded in becoming one of the most defining voices in modern psychology. Talk about not squandering your suffering.

Given her lived experience, it's no wonder Linehan set out to transform psychotherapy when she was in a position to do so. In the remainder of this chapter, I'll discuss the science and philosophy that also informed Linehan's perspective on validation. I'll then share DBT's validation skills and briefly discuss how I've adapted them. Most important, I'm going to try to tie all of this back to *you* and your suffering. I know I've already made a lot of points about how validation transforms lives, but I want to close part 1 with one more: **The greatest gift that comes from knowing how to validate others is the opportunity to find meaning in suffering.**

---

sophisticated in my humor and want to leave you with the image of her distracting Carl Rogers with a cat toy while stuffing papers from his desk into an alligator purse.

A couple of notes before we proceed:

1. The upcoming discussion about the science of psychotherapies might not seem terribly relevant to non-therapists. If, however, you replace the word *therapist* with *parent, manager, spouse,* or anyone else trying to effect change, the relevance becomes apparent. As the late, great Carl Rogers said, "An atmosphere of acceptance and respect, of deep understanding, is a good climate for personal growth, and as such applies to children, colleagues, students, as well as [therapy] clients."[1]

2. Most people don't finish books these days. You're about a quarter of the way through this one, which means you've reached the point when many (myself included) abandon their books. I can't help but worry that the promise of science and philosophy might push you over the "I'll come back to this later" line. If that's the case, you can skip this section and go straight to "I Think Your Work on Validation Was Groundbreaking." I wouldn't recommend skipping it, though, because you'll miss out on dialectics, which I reference throughout the book and is the all-time best excuse for contradicting yourself.

"I STOLE THAT FROM CARL ROGERS"

The Science: Western Psychology

Carl Rogers was an interesting character. In 1957, he published a now-legendary paper[2] suggesting that any improvements a person achieves through therapy result from their therapist's genuineness, empathy, and acceptance.* That's it. Want to help someone become more assertive? Accept them. Want them to scream

---

* Rogers used the term *unconditional positive regard* to describe the combination of genuineness, empathy, and acceptance.

less and smile more? Accept them. Rogers rejected the views of be-haviorists like B. F. Skinner, who believed that change has more to do with reinforcements and punishments than self-discovery.[3] He also took issue with the holier-than-thou attitude in Freud's psy-choanalytic therapy, which was all the rage at the time.[4] The as-sumption that doctors are superior to their patients—which was rampant in psychoanalysis—was outright toxic as far as Rogers was concerned. Disappointed by the state of his field, Rogers devel-oped his own therapy approach.[5] He cautioned therapists against pushing for change and discouraged interpretation and analysis.[6] I cannot emphasize enough what a giant middle finger his work was to the prevailing theories of the time. I mean, it was an empathic and accepting middle finger, but a middle finger nonetheless.

Despite being a fierce advocate of clinical research, Rogers abruptly left academia in the early 1960s, and research on the ther-apy he developed began petering out. In retrospect, it seems Rog-ers was right that acceptance, empathy, and understanding create a good "climate" for individual growth. Unfortunately, he didn't offer many techniques to help therapists establish this climate. And he'd failed to appreciate that although acceptance can inspire important changes, it often needs to be used alongside, not in place of, behavioral change strategies like skills training and posi-tive reinforcement.

By the time Linehan came on the scene, behavioral and cog-nitive behavioral therapies had become the gold standard. Although they'd grown increasingly egalitarian and collaborative—thanks to Rogers's influence on the field—Linehan found their emphasis on change was often problematic, particularly when people were resistant to it: "'You're not listening to me.' 'You're trying to change me,'" she wrote in her memoir, recalling what clients said when she attempted to help them develop new skills or problem-solve.[7] She experimented with going full-on Rogerian, focusing on accep-tance rather than change, but it didn't work, "'What? You're not going to help me?' the client would say. 'You're just going to leave me here, in all this pain?'"[8] By this point, I imagine Linehan was running out of chapters in her *How to Be a Therapist* textbook. Despite the setbacks, she remained convinced that acceptance was a meaningful piece of the therapy puzzle. In need of a new direction, Linehan took to the streets to learn everything she could about acceptance. And by streets, I mean Buddhist monasteries.

The Philosophy: Zen Buddhism and Dialectics

The transformative effects of acceptance are emphasized across all sects of Buddhism. Realizing she needed to deepen her understanding of acceptance, Linehan took a hiatus from academia to live at Shasta Abbey—a Zen monastery in California.[9] From there, she headed to Germany, where she studied under a Zen master. I imagine Linehan's immersion into Eastern philosophy as a fast-action movie montage. Pan to her sitting in meditation, then reading ancient scripture by candlelight, then wringing her hands in frustration before finally opening her palms in acceptance. After almost a year of throwing herself into Zen Buddhism, Linehan returned to work on DBT with a better understanding of acceptance and how to balance it with behaviorism.

In the end, the validation skills she developed allowed therapists to communicate acceptance in ways that resonated with clients and made them more receptive to change. They offered pathways to the genuineness, acceptance, and empathy that Rogers espoused, which increased the success of the behavioral interventions Skinner inspired.

The approach of synthesizing opposite positions like acceptance and change reflects the dialectical mindset that is DBT's namesake. The "dialectical" in Dialectical Behavior Therapy refers to the synthesis of opposing ideas.[10] It's a philosophical form of reasoning that can be used to challenge black-or-white thinking—the obnoxious, photoshop-like filter our minds insist on applying to reality. Black-or-white thinking allows us to make snap judgments so we can quickly navigate our environment (e.g., stick with the "good" berries, avoid the "bad" mushrooms) but it also distorts reality.

Dialectics replaces the "either/or" with a "both/and" perspective, allowing for the coexistence of opposites. For example, a person can be both good *and* bad, both weak *and* strong. Not only does the dialectical framework introduce a new "reality"—the person who is both good and bad is categorically different from someone who is only one or the other—but it's also presumed to draw one closer to the "the truth" because reality is more nuanced than our black-or-white thinking would have us believe.

Although dialectics proved to be transformative for clients, I suspect Linehan incorporated the philosophy into her treatment so she'd have a "Get Out of Jail Free" card when she contradicted herself: "You said you accept me as I am." Linehan: "I do." "Then why are you saying I need to do more, try harder, and be more motivated to change?" Linehan: "Because that's also true." "That's bullshit." Linehan: "That's dialectics." Mic dropped.

As you work on developing the skills in this book, you'll find that validation is in many ways an exercise in dialectics. Looking for the kernel of truth in another person's perspective, especially when so much of it seems "bad," helps you see the reality between the black-and-white extremes your mind prefers. You will have to be more intentional about challenging your judgments. You can't just write off someone as a jerk. Instead, you have to figure out what's reasonable or valid in the jerk's perspective, which will inevitably challenge your conclusion that they're just a jerk.

It is easier to rely on judgments, but it's also more painful. Fear and anger toward the "bad," self-loathing, and disappointment from failing to be "good" enough are the costs of lizard-braining through life. Fortunately, there's another way. A middle path that exists between the extremes. It's not the route we're naturally drawn toward, but it's one you can grow accustomed to taking.

"I THINK YOUR WORK ON VALIDATION WAS GROUNDBREAKING"

DBT's Levels of Validation are what ultimately helped me transform my innate sensitivity into something of a superpower.[11] The levels consist of six skills arranged in order of strength. According to Linehan, each level is more complete and depends on the one(s) before it.[12]

Level 1. Pay attention: Listen, observe, and look interested.

Level 2. Reflect back: Restate what the person said to you in a nonjudgmental tone.

Level 3. Read minds: Communicate what else you think a person might be experiencing based on what they've disclosed.

Level 4. Understand/communicate an understanding of the causes: Acknowledge past experiences and other factors that might be contributing to someone's reaction.

Level 5. Acknowledge the valid: Communicate that you consider someone's behavior, emotions, or thoughts to be valid given the current facts of the situation.

Level 6. Show equality: Act authentically, treating the other person with respect and as an equal. Refrain from saying or doing anything that suggests you are above them.

You might look at that list and think, "Nothing new here. I do this stuff all the time." I have a similar experience whenever I see a new recipe. I think, "I know how to whisk eggs and ice." Pan to me two hours later when I'm frantically calling grocery stores to see if they have a *Moana*-themed birthday cake in stock to replace the Pinterest fail that's sitting in my garbage. The moral is, don't underestimate the importance of technique, timing, and training when it comes to validation—or baking, for that matter.

Part 2 employs the method used in clinical training programs of combining basic instruction, real-life examples, and practical exercises to help you quickly and reliably develop validation skills. Even though I'll give you what amounts to clinical training, it won't be challenging or academic. I teach these skills as I experience them—through movie clips and quotes, anecdotes of breakthroughs, and the occasional breakdown. My goal is to draw your attention to what's already there, turning up the volume on a language that's all around us but rarely spoken loudly or consistently enough for one to become proficient in it.

Although the skills you'll be learning were developed for DBT, I've never reserved them for DBT clients. I have yet to experience a form of suffering that could not be decreased by attending to others, and I know of no better method by which to do so than validation. During the years, I've adapted, expanded, and recontextualized the validation skills in DBT to make them more accessible and applicable outside of therapy. But before turning to my approach to these skills, I want to make good on the promise to tie this all back to your suffering. To do so, I need to reiterate a point I just made: I have yet to experience a form of suffering that could not be decreased by attending to others.

"YOUR SUFFERING IS A GIFT; DON'T SQUANDER IT"

I have suffered a lot in my life. Maybe not more than you, or that guy over there, but I'm no stranger to suffering. And neither are you. It doesn't matter who you are, where you come from, or where you end up; you will suffer. My disease might be your divorce, unemployment, failure to launch, estrangement from family, ineptitude, or other experience that culminates in suffering.

The Zen master Thich Nhat Hanh described suffering as the mud that gives rise to lotus flowers. No mud, no flowers.[13] But in my experience, suffering doesn't always pay dividends. More often than not, it just leads to more suffering. Once he was liberated from Auschwitz, after having spent three years in various concentration camps, clinician Viktor Frankl published a book, *Man's Search for Meaning*, based on the notes he took while living in the death camps. In it, he makes some bold declarations about suffering. Put simply, he said the question of what suffering does to us is a matter of what we do with it. Do we create meaning from it? Do we connect with others through it? If so, we can thrive. If not, we might not survive. According to Frankl, "despair is suffering without meaning."[14] All mud, no flowers.

Frankl's perspective echoes Zen Buddhist philosophy, which suggests that suffering is not meant to be avoided, but confronted. Not endured, but transformed. In the words of Thich Nhat Hanh, "When we learn to acknowledge, embrace, and understand our suffering, we suffer much less. Not only that, but we're also able to go further and transform our suffering into understanding, compassion, and joy for ourselves and for others."[15]

I'd seen that awareness, understanding, and empathy were the by-products of my innate sensitivity and the depression I experienced earlier in my life. The validation skills I mastered allowed me to channel these experiences in ways that helped others grow and brought meaning to my life. By the time I met Linehan, I'd loosely connected these dots in my head. But I'd not said any of this out loud.

I'd also never considered my physical illness to be a source of pain and suffering that could come to have meaning in the way my depression had—by allowing me to better understand and validate others. I associated terms like *pain* and *suffering* with the mental anguish I'd experienced from depression. I was in my twenties when I was diagnosed with MS, and I didn't have any colleagues or friends with chronic medical conditions. At least, none that I knew of. The first supervisors I told about my disease advised me against disclosing it to my clients. "You don't want them to feel like they have to take care of you," one insisted. "They must see you as competent and capable if they're going to trust you," said another.

Confined to hiding what was becoming a central part of my daily life, I soon found myself in the familiar territory of believing that nobody else could possibly understand what I was going through. The stepchild of that thought was the belief that my disease distanced me from others. I saw it as a liability, not an asset. I'd unknowingly slotted MS into the category of "bad," having failed to consider the dialectical perspective that it could be used for "good."

After meeting with Linehan, I decided not to abandon my ambitions of becoming a DBT therapist. I did, however, accept that I needed to make some changes. I wasn't going to be able to see DBT clients full-time. I cut short my fellowship to start a private practice in which I could determine my own hours, caseload, and curfew. I began supervising students for Linehan, a gig she kindly allowed me to maintain after I moved to California.

Most important, our conversation during the retreat brought into sharp focus the blurry lines I'd connected between suffering, validation, and meaning. I realized that pain doesn't need to be neatly resolved or in the distant past for us to use it constructively. If anything, it's the other way around—using our suffering to help us better connect with others *is* how to use it constructively. We might need to learn how to temper or tolerate suffering so that we can fully attend to others, but this in and of itself is therapeutic.

When it was unclear if my mom would survive or be able to function after her brain surgery, I realized how much more devastating and confusing these circumstances would have been if, like my client Ella who lost her mom at a young age, I'd had to face them as a child. How could I communicate the greater awareness, understanding, and empathy I had for Ella's experience without making it all about me or suggesting that what I was going through as an adult in any way compared to the loss she'd endured as a child? Which validation skills could I use to thread that needle? These were the questions I returned to when hopelessness and concern for my mom overwhelmed me. The belief that their answers might bring relief to someone else helped me confront parts of my experience I otherwise would have avoided. When everything about the situation with my mom seemed wrong, focusing on what my experience might teach me about Ella's was one of the few things that felt right.

Similarly, when I felt the familiar pangs of "mom guilt" after taking a break from Havana when she was sick, I recalled how validated I'd felt when parents shared similar parenting struggles with me. Then I thought of all the other caregivers beating themselves up for the fatigue they mistake for selfishness and wondered if disclosing my inner struggle might help validate someone else's. Despite my instincts, I initially decided against including my story in this book. "Who am I to think that my parenting concerns matter or might help someone?" I thought. Then I reflected on the more important question: Why should I conclude that they can't?

The US Surgeon General Vivek Murthy declared that we are in an "epidemic of loneliness."[16] Nothing degrades people more than feeling unseen and unheard. Mindfulness, understanding, and empathy are the fruits of our suffering; validation allows us to use those fruits to nourish others who are starving. I'm not saying that you must deeply suffer in order to effectively validate someone or that validation pertains only to negative emotions. The point is simply that in exercising these skills, you will come to appreciate not only the validity in your own struggles but the utility in them as well.

While scouring the DBT research, I did not find a single article on how validating others affects one's own mental health or quality of life. And yet when I reviewed the history of modern psychology and the philosophies that influenced it, this seems like a pretty obvious conclusion. In fact, I think there are several meaningful conclusions that can be drawn from all these perspectives, and they summarize the main points of this chapter nicely:

1. It is possible to accept people *and* help them change. The principles of behaviorism are one piece of this puzzle. Validation skills are another.

2. We're judgmental by nature. Your judgments won't magically go away, but with practice, you can get better at noticing and reframing them. Challenging instinct with intention is how character is formed.

3. It's possible to both resist *and* embrace suffering. When approached in this way—with a tenacious spirit to fight against it and an eye toward the awareness, understanding, empathy, and acceptance it inspires—suffering can be channeled into meaning.

Having discussed what validation is, why it's important, and where it came from, we turn now to the next obvious question. How do you validate people?

PART 2

HOW

CHAPTER 5

THE VALIDATION LADDER— EIGHT STEPS TO SEEING AND BEING SEEN

Skill to do comes of doing.
—RALPH WALDO EMERSON, *THE ATLANTIC*

This chapter is like an instruction manual for the rest of the chapters in part 2. It provides an overview of the Validation Ladder, my model of validation, which includes eight skills you can use to communicate it. The remaining chapters in this part zoom in on each skill individually. Although I'll provide detailed instruction on how to have success with these skills, external factors like social norms, political climate, one's culture, and power dynamics often have the final say on what will or will not be effective. If your sense of what's appropriate in a situation conflicts with something I've said, trust your gut.

Understanding the model and the skills is important. Having said that, I'll now do my dialectical thing and tell you not to worry if this information doesn't immediately click for you. Oprah, Jon Stewart, Terry Gross—these people became validation all-stars without ever studying the skills you'll be learning. In the examples I provide of these three in action, you'll see that they rely heavily on the skills in this book. They just never formally studied them. At least, not as far as I know. Instead, they acquired these skills unknowingly through the hundreds of hours they spent in their high-stakes careers trying to validate others. I don't doubt these icons are all emotionally intelligent, but that alone would not have made them the validation superstars they are today. They had the feedback of live audiences and the media to reinforce them when they were effective, allowing them to develop their skills without even realizing it. And they had a "show must go on" mandate to prevent them from giving up when they erred along the way.

I make this point because you're about to get a crash course in validation. Everything the all-stars learned through exhaustive trial and error can be found in part 2. But when it comes to validating your kid on the heels of their first heartbreak or your sister after she calls off her engagement, you need to be in the moment, not in your head. When I train therapists and clients in validation, I give them the same information I'll share with you in these pages. Then, at the end of the training, I tell them to ignore everything they learned and just focus on validating people. I encourage you to do the same. Your intention with validation is always to "Show that you're there, you get it, and you care." When in doubt, rely on this simple mantra to point you in the direction of validation and back to the skills you learned to communicate it.

SHOW THAT YOU'RE THERE, YOU GET IT, AND YOU CARE.

Before we go any farther, the therapist in me wants to be sure you're fully informed about what's to come. Part 2 focuses on validating *others*. Side effects from reading these chapters may include thinking people in your life need this book more than you because they suck at validation, daydreaming about people validating you, feeling guilty about daydreaming about people validating you when you're supposed to be learning how to validate others, and remembering that the author said something about how validation leads to change and wishing she'd get to that part already. Side effects are to be expected, so please don't judge yourself if you experience them. And although it helps to be aware of possible side effects, I hope they won't deter you. You must approach acceptance as an end in and of itself if it is to become a means to change.

THE VALIDATION LADDER

Models are inherently abstract and occasionally yawn-inducing, so I promise to keep this section brief and include illustrations whenever possible.

Three Skill Sets

Validation shows that you accept another person's experience as valid through the mindfulness, understanding, and empathy you demonstrate. The Validation Ladder includes three subsets of skills designed to help you communicate these qualities (see illustration 1). Each section of the ladder represents one of the three skill sets. The **Mindfulness Skills** at the bottom typically convey subtle forms of validation but are very accessible; the **Empathy Skills** at the top are super validating but can be trickier to pull off. And the **Understanding Skills** in the middle—well, they're somewhere in between the Mindfulness and Empathy skills. When I talk about the strength and difficulty of these skill sets, I'm speaking in generalities. The **Empathy Skills** are generally perceived as more impactful than the **Understanding Skills**, which are generally more impactful than the **Mindfulness Skills**. There are exceptions to this rule,* but on average, that's how they shake out.

Each skill set builds off the previous one(s) and achieves its aims: the **Understanding Skills** require and communicate mindfulness and understanding, and the **Empathy Skills** demonstrate mindfulness, understanding, and empathy, which is why they're so powerful. Although the **Understanding Skills** and **Empathy Skills** may be more validating, you never want to fake understanding or concern. When it comes to validation, authenticity is critical to success. You might have to go outside of your comfort zone from time to time while practicing validation, but you never want to say things you don't believe.

---

* You'll find one such exception in chapter 6, where I explain how magician Derek DelGaudio masterfully validated an entire live audience using only the Mindfulness Skills.

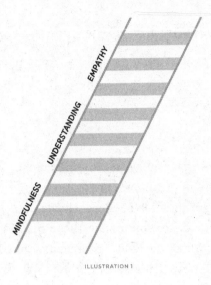

ILLUSTRATION 1

Now for my favorite thing about the Validation Ladder: in addition to communicating mindfulness, the **Mindfulness Skills** double as tools for developing understanding and empathy, and in addition to demonstrating understanding, the **Understanding Skills** help you further generate empathy. Each skill set makes it easier to access the one(s) above it. The relationship between these skill sets speaks to the nature of mindfulness, understanding, and empathy in general. Nonjudgmental observation leads to insight, which fosters emotional connection.

Eight Skills

The skills in the Validation Ladder allow you to validate what you genuinely consider valid, while simultaneously fostering deeper levels of acceptance. There are eight skills in total—two mindfulness, three understanding, and three empathy (see illustration 2). Together, the skills in the Validation Ladder form the acronym ACCEPTED, which is how people will feel if you're effective in using them. Note that the skills in each skill set are not listed in order of strength. Each *set* of skills is generally more potent than the one before it, but the skills in each set are more or less interchangeable.

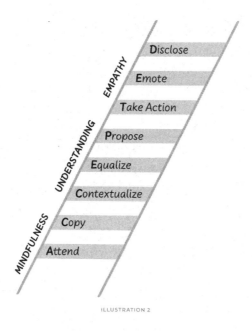

ILLUSTRATION 2

LEARNING IS A SCIENCE

You don't have to rely on learning principles to write a book, but you do if you want people to retain and apply the information it contains. I want to highlight two of the principles I relied on while crafting this book because you can use them yourself to master the skills in the Validation Ladder.

The first principle is that repetition fosters learning. As you may have deduced from the seventeen times I have reiterated the definition of validation, I repeat myself. A lot. I do it because repetition is one of the easiest ways to help you passively absorb information. But to convert this information into behavioral skills, you'll need to apply it. Neuroscience has shown that repeating skills results in long-term potentiation—the strengthening of neural connections in the brain. The stronger these connections are, the faster they fire; the faster they fire, the more automated the skills associated with them become. Eventually, performing the skill requires little thought or effort.

When I teach validation, I introduce one skill at a time and have folks practice that skill for a week before presenting the next one.* At the end of eight weeks, I tell them to simply make a point of validating people. That's it. In my experience, this method of zooming in on each skill and then zooming out to focus on the objective (validating) is the most successful way of teaching validation, and I encourage you to use it as you move through part 2. At the end of each skills chapter, you'll find tips on how to practice that skill during the week. After you've practiced each skill individually, you can focus on just your objective—validating someone—rather than the mechanics of what you're doing.

The second principle I want to highlight is that we learn by watching others. The approach of teaching through demonstration is known as modeling, and it has proven critical to helping people develop new behaviors. With interpersonal skills, modeling works best when it's organic. A real-life example of someone using a skill is more instructive than a made-up one in which everything goes according to plan.

Modeling skills is obviously challenging for an author, but I have some workarounds. The first is to include anecdotes from my personal life and work as a therapist, which you're probably used to me doing by now. The second is to rely on examples from the media, and the third is to have you keep an eye out for others using these skills as you learn them.

Don't worry if you can't identify with my therapy examples or aren't familiar with the media excerpts I include; instead, focus on identifying the skills in play. These skills really are all around us. Your task is to become increasingly mindful of when people use them and use them well. Also, if you happen to find an exemplary example of validation, feel free to email me via back channels through my website. I collect validation examples like wealthy people collect fine art.

---

* Two of the skills, Attending and Proposing, can benefit from more repetition than you can usually get in one week. I'll discuss how to drill these skills when we come to them.

WHEN YOU MESS UP

Anyone who makes a habit of practicing validation will strike out now and then. In general, the more validating a skill has the potential to be if it succeeds, the more punishing it will feel if it fails. **As with any ladder, the higher you go, the harder the fall.** Although mistakes can be painful, you should never assume defeat after failing to communicate a high level of validation. Instead, just return to the **Mindfulness Skills** and focus on being present. Usually, when our attempts to convey a higher level of validation go sideways, it's because we haven't been listening closely.

If you study someone—a coach, colleague, mentor, or spouse—who seems to have a knack for validation, you'll see that they don't actually make every shot they take. They just don't get distracted or discouraged when their attempts fail.

I remember watching an episode of *Oprah* back in graduate school when I was trying to perfect my validation game and being surprised by two things: (1) how many different ways Oprah tried to validate someone in a single guest interview and (2) how often she failed. A typical interview would go something like this: the guest describes a challenging moment in their life, and Oprah says something like, "That must have been frustrating." The guest responds with a correction: "It wasn't frustrating. It was terrifying." Oprah takes a step back without missing a beat despite having whiffed her validation attempt in front of a live studio audience: "Terrifying. What was terrifying about it?" She listens thoughtfully and maybe follows up once or twice to clarify something they said or repeat it to them. Then she steps it up again, offering some insight they hadn't articulated and checking to see if it resonates. She might need to do this several times, but eventually, she nails it. The guest nods their head in response to her deft validation and begins to tear up as Oprah takes their hand in hers. The camera pans to the audience; there's not a dry eye in the place. Everyone has been Oprahfied. What stands out in Oprah's interviews isn't the times when she fails; it's the impact she has when she succeeds.

I'm warning you now that despite how unshakable pros like Oprah appear, it can hurt when people are unresponsive or put off by your attempts to validate them. When this happens, remember that validation isn't about you (unless you're validating yourself); it's about bringing mindful awareness, understanding, and empathy to another person's experience so that they feel accepted. Don't let your ego distract you from your goal. Taking in feedback and adjusting your approach are validating in their own right. **Most everyone will appreciate the opportunity to be heard by someone who is genuinely trying to listen.**

I also should mention the other, perhaps higher-stake risk you take when attempting to validate someone: exposing yourself to invalidation in the process. Climbing the Validation Ladder requires you to reveal more of your authentic self. The **Mindfulness Skills** at the bottom show that you're paying attention; you don't reveal much, so there's not much for the other person to invalidate at this level. Moving up to the **Understanding Skills** requires you to share your thoughts. Now things start to get personal. Any thoughts you express could be invalidated, which might sting. Last week, I was at the park with Havana and struck up a conversation with a nanny who said she was working two full-time nannying gigs while tending to her ailing husband. "You must feel like you're always caring for people," I said to validate her. When she exasperatedly exclaimed, "No, I don't!" I didn't just feel like an idiot; I felt rejected. I wanted to cut and run. Instead, I went back to using the **Mindfulness Skills** until I felt more confident in my understanding to try again. We eventually overcame what I soon realized was a language barrier. Still, I'd be lying if I said her reaction to my initial validation attempt didn't sting.

To pull off the **Empathy Skills** at the top of the Validation Ladder, you've got to be even more vulnerable. In addition to revealing your thoughts, these skills require you to share your resources, emotions, and experiences. The personal nature of the **Empathy Skills** is what makes them so impactful. It's also what makes them so risky. In the coming chapters, I'll discuss the risks associated with the higher validation skills and offer ways to manage them. For now, I'll just add that with great risk comes great reward. Not only do the higher skill sets enable you to validate others more deeply, they also allow you to experience higher levels of validation in return.

RECAP

The Validation Ladder consists of three skill sets used to communicate varying degrees of validation. There are a total of eight validation skills among these three skill sets. Practicing as you go and keeping an eye out for people using these skills are the best strategies you can use to master them quickly. You'll find that skills higher up the Validation Ladder are more likely to communicate *in*validation when executed poorly; when done well, they're also more likely to result in reciprocal validation—wherein both you and the person you're validating feel seen. We turn now to the first set of skills in the Validation Ladder: the *magical* **Mindfulness Skills**.

CHAPTER 6

ATTEND—THE GAME ALL GOOD LISTENERS PLAY

The greatest compliment that was ever paid to me was when one
asked me what I thought, and attended to my answer.
—HENRY DAVID THOREAU, "LIFE WITHOUT PRINCIPLE"

"Please take this moment to turn off your phones and silence any distractions. Thank you for your attention." These words appear on the screen at the beginning of *In and Of Itself*, the film adaptation of Derek DelGaudio's live theater performance by the same name. The film splices together scenes from the magic show he performed more than five hundred times in three years.

DelGaudio is a distinctly uncharismatic entertainer. His voice is monotone, his movements are restrained, and, as one attendee noted, "He has sad eyes." About three-quarters of the way through his show, DelGaudio asks an audience member how they think it will end. The film highlights various answers people have given among his many performances. One person says there will be a flash of light, and DelGaudio will be replaced by an elephant. Another poetically predicts that "Everyone will find love. No one will feel judged. Our 'I ams,' will become 'we are.'" When I heard that I was like, "This dude has clearly never been to a magic show." Today I'm convinced that he was either a psychic or a repeat customer because he nailed it. DelGaudio achieves the impossible right before our eyes, but not through defying our expectations of the physical world by, say, sawing someone in half or making an elephant appear out of thin air. Instead, he transcends the limits of communication and relationships, using validation as his sleight of hand. The effect is nothing short of magical. By the end of DelGaudio's final trick, I felt seen, accepted, and valued, despite being alone, in the dark, in my pajamas. I'll show you how DelGaudio works his validation magic, but first, I have to describe his seminal trick. If you read closely, you might be able to catch the ten to fifteen things he says and does to deftly validate the audience.

The film begins with footage from the lobby, where audience members are arriving for the show. We see them milling around a brightly lit wall with hundreds of cards hanging from it. The tops of the cards are all the same; they say: "I AM." The bottoms are different and include descriptions like "a feminist," "a good time," "a teacher." Each person is asked to pick a card from the wall and then hand it to an usher before entering the theater. The cards aren't referenced again until the end of the show, when DelGaudio glances at the pile of collected cards that has appeared onstage. Without reading or touching them, he turns to the audience. He asks anyone who picked a card because it described how they truly see themselves to stand up. Most everyone does.

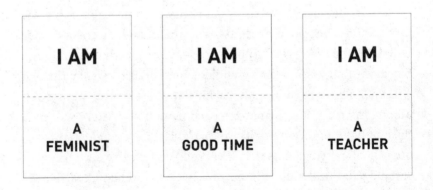

He continues: "I remember reading that true identity . . . is that which exists within one's own heart and is seen by another. Honestly, I have no idea if that's true outside these walls these days, but in here"—he locks eyes with someone in the first row—"I see a bartender." The man in the first row cracks what can only be described as a "shut the front door" smile. How did DelGaudio know he'd chosen the "I am a bartender" card?! DelGaudio's gaze moves to the woman standing next to the bartender guy. "A curiosity," he says, and gets another look of surprise following another correct *guess*. A slight shift from his robotic tone introduces some levity as he declares that an older woman with glasses is, in fact, "a midnight toker."

During the next fifteen minutes, DelGaudio correctly "guesses" each person's card. "A lover, an alchemist, a truth-teller," he says as his eyes flash from person to person. With each correct answer, the momentum seems to build. People become visibly moved by his words, *their* words. He is just repeating the descriptions they chose for themselves.

"A Good Samaritan," he says to an older gentleman with glasses. The man's hand flies to his mouth, where it trembles uncontrollably as he fights back tears. People aren't just watching DelGaudio by this point; they're looking at each other, nodding, sharing smiles, even reaching over the aisles to tenderly squeeze each other's shoulders.

"A vegan, a good time, a feminist." He pauses for a second and nods slightly before calling out "an achiever" while locking eyes with a woman as though personally confirming that this is the case. Just when you start to suspect that all of the people in the audience are plants, paid to act surprised and get teary, he happens upon Bill Gates. "A leader," DelGaudio declares. Gates offers a wry smile before sitting down.

The emotional climax occurs halfway through the trick when DelGaudio turns to a man who has the type of desperate, faraway look that breaks this therapist's heart. DelGaudio puts his hands on his hips. He focuses on the man for several seconds, which feels more like minutes, before looking down and closing his eyes. Then he lifts his head, fixing his gaze once more on the man staring back at him in anticipation. DelGaudio starts to speak but then stops, as if whatever word this man chose to describe himself is too painful to acknowledge out loud. Finally, he says it: "A nobody." The man maintains eye contact with the magician while folding his arms across his chest to hug himself. His eyes soften and twinkle with wetness as he sits back down. Tears are reflected in DelGaudio's eyes as well. Oddly, this moment doesn't feel intrusive or exploitative. It feels tender, supportive, even loving.

Initially, DelGaudio calls out people's card descriptions from the stage. Then he moves into the aisles. Eventually, he makes his way into the rows, where he stands face-to-face with audience members while reciting the words they chose to describe themselves.

DelGaudio is essentially performing two tricks simultaneously. I have no idea how he pulls off the first one, correctly guessing the cards each person selected before entering the theater. This trick is impressive, but it doesn't result in the "seeing/being seen" effect that defines the show. For that "trick," he relies almost exclusively on the **Mindfulness Skills**—Attending and Copying. At the beginning of the show, he asked viewers to give him their full attention; he achieves the powerful effect of his final "trick" by giving them his.

I put *trick* in quotation marks above because there is no real trickery, deception, or illusion behind what he's doing. As you know, validation works only if it's sincere. Even magicians can't escape this constraint. "That moment of watching people be and feel really, *genuinely* seen is the magic of the show," DelGaudio said in an interview with *GQ* magazine.[1] "It's all leading up to that single moment of another person looking at another person and just going, 'I see you, man. I see you standing there. I know who you are. I totally get you. In this moment, I see all of you.' And that is like a fuckin' gift that we struggle to receive every single day. And because we're all struggling to receive it, we forget to give it."

In the coming pages, I'll show you how DelGaudio gives the gift of being seen to a theater full of strangers using the **Mindfulness Skills**—Attending and Copying. More important, I'll explain everything you need to know to experience the magic of these skills firsthand. This chapter covers Attending—what it is and how you, like DelGaudio, can use it to validate people without saying a word.

ATTENDING 101

In a sentence, Attending means paying attention and listening without judgment in a way that shows interest and cultivates understanding.* Attending conveys that you are "there"—physically, emotionally, and mentally—and that the other person is worthy of your attention, a subtle but powerful message.

In physics, the "observer effect" refers to the disturbance that results from observation.[2] By observing and measuring things like thermal energy or electrons, we change how they behave. A series of studies in psychology between 1924 and 1932 showed that a similar effect occurs in human interactions. In what came to be known as the Hawthorne effect, researchers found that when people knew they were being observed, they changed their behavior.[3]

The finding that people act differently when they know they're being watched wouldn't make for a clickable headline these days. What continues to captivate us, though, is the magnitude of these effects. In 2010, South African filmmaker Craig Foster developed an unlikely bond with an octopus by visiting her every day for one

---

* Other names for Attending include Paying Attention, Active Listening, Deep Listening, Mindful Listening, and Listening and Observing. These skills are all more or less synonymous with each other. (Marsha M. Linehan, *DBT Skills Training Handouts and Worksheets*, 2nd ed., "Interpersonal Effectiveness Handout 18: A 'How To' Guide to Validation" [New York: Guilford Publications, 2014]; Kathryn R. Robertson, "Active Listening: More than Just Paying Attention," *PubMed* 34, no. 12 [December 1, 2005]: 1053–55, https://pubmed.ncbi.nlm.nih.gov/16333490; Julia Ziemer, "Deep Listening: To Understand a Different Perspective," *LSE* [blog], June 25, 2020, https://blogs.lse.ac.uk/socialbusinesshub/2020/06/25/deep-listening-to-understand-a-different-perspective; MasterClass, "Mindful Listening Benefits: 5 Ways to Practice Mindful Listening—2023—MasterClass," *MasterClass Articles*, August 19, 2021, https://www.masterclass.com/articles/mindful-listening-guide; Marsha M. Linehan, "Validation and Psychotherapy," in *Empathy Reconsidered: New Directions in Psychotherapy*, eds. A. C. Bohart and L. S. Greenberg [Washington, DC: American Psychological Association, 1997], 360, https://doi.org/10.1037/10226-016.)

year in her natural habitat, the kelp forest. Although she initially cowered in fear when he approached, she slowly began to seek him out, eventually clinging to his chest and allowing him to hold her. They never exchanged words, obviously, and Foster didn't rely on any octopus treats to win her over. Their relationship was established and nourished through observation alone. "I fell in love with her, but also with that amazing 'wildness' that she represents and how that changed me."[4] Foster's documentary *My Octopus Teacher*, which shared his footage from this period, became an international sensation, earning the Academy Award for Best Documentary Feature.[5] I'm not saying you should expect to win an Oscar for Attending, but if you did, it wouldn't be the first time such a thing happened.

Attending's ability to forge connections isn't specific to human-octopus relationships. Showing up is the language of intimacy. Do you RSVP to that party? Watch from the stands when your kids have a game? Offer to accompany a friend to their first AA meeting? Nonjudgmentally bearing witness to the experiences that shape a person's life is the most direct way to validate their significance. These easy-to-dismiss moments can determine crucial features of our relationships, including whether or not we have them at all.

Inattention, on the other hand, deprives our relationships of the nutrients they need to thrive; it's also a swift way to invalidate others and is frequently weaponized for these purposes. Just watch politicians during a debate. Rather than following along or jotting down notes in response to something their opponent said, many make a point of looking bored or distracted. They have weird little side conversations with people off-camera or become *really* fixated on straightening their pins. Russian president Vladimir Putin favors slouching and sleepy eyes, giving the impression that he's struggling to stay awake. He's so over the top, you'd think he was acting out a charades prompt that reads "listening to someone who is unworthy of your attention."

It's not simply that paying attention to people, or octopuses in

Foster's case, is good and ignoring them is bad. It wouldn't feel validating if someone were glaring and giving you the middle finger as you delivered a speech. **For your attention to read as validating, it must convey interest and nonjudgment.** Being able to reliably do this regardless of who is across from you—or attending your magic show—takes skill.

HOW TO ATTEND

I hate being the bearer of bad news, but paying attention and demonstrating that you're paying attention are not the same thing. The former is a cognitive process; the latter is an interpersonal skill. Even if you remain nonjudgmental and genuinely interested in someone, your attention won't ascend to the level of validation if it's not perceived as such. To consistently clear the Attending bar, you need to use nonverbals, listen, and ask questions and comment.

Use Nonverbals
More commonly known as body language, nonverbals include physical *behaviors* like nodding and eye contact, as well as *vocal cues* like volume, pitch, speed, and simple utterances such as "Uh-huh," "Yeah," and "Hmm." I'll discuss vocal cues more in a moment.

When it comes to nonverbal behaviors, some are better than others at communicating engagement. Fortunately, researchers have been geeking out on this stuff for years and have developed a sophisticated understanding of which nonverbals are most effective at signaling attention, connection, and safety. They refer to these nonverbals as "immediacy behaviors," so-called because they reduce the psychological and physical distance between people.[6] I've narrowed them down to the Big Four: *

---

* Cultural norms may influence how nonverbals are interpreted. Maintaining eye contact, for instance, is considered more important in Western European than East Asian countries and may even be perceived as disrespectful in some cultures. When in doubt, take your cues from the other person and follow their lead. (David Matsumoto and Hyi Sung Hwang, "Cultural Influences on Nonverbal Behavior," in *Nonverbal Communication: Science and Applications*, eds., Mark G. Frank and Hyi Sung Hwang [Thousand Oaks,

1. Eye contact
2. Proximity (standing close or leaning in)
3. Gesturing
4. Nodding[7]

Throughout his performance, DelGaudio's use of the Big Four is masterful. In the trick I described, he relies exclusively on *eye contact* (#1) to communicate who he's focusing on. At various points, he allows his gaze to linger on someone for several seconds before speaking, which draws out the time he spends looking at them, seeing them. Moving in closer *proximity* (#2) to the audience allows him to safely and steadily increase the sense of intimacy during the course of the trick, while *gesturing* (#3) and *nodding* (#4) deftly draw out audience members' reactions. He crosses his arms; they raise an eyebrow. He nods in affirmation (#4); they nod back. The more he engages with people in this way, the more they engage with each other—not by talking, but through these basic immediacy behaviors.

Anyone who incorporates the Big Four is capable of achieving similar results. Using them in concert, as DelGaudio does, can amplify their effects, culminating in a powerful signal of validation that captures people's attention and opens their hearts. Note that you don't need to be dramatic with the Big Four for them to be effective. You might deliberately look up from your phone to show that you're listening, but you don't need to make a production out of it. **The key to being natural is to be intentional about what you're doing without focusing too much on how it looks.**

CA: SAGE Publications, 2013], 97–120; Shota Uono and Jari K. Hietanen, "Eye Contact Perception in the West and East: A Cross-Cultural Study," *PLOS One* 10, no. 2 [February 25, 2015]: e0118094, https://doi.org/10.1371/journal.pone.0118094.)

Listen

Listening entails more than just shutting up and giving the other person a chance to talk. If you're thinking about what you will say next or trying to decide if you can get away with eating pizza for the third night in a row, you're not listening. You're just being quiet. Listening demands your undivided attention. Attending (listening to validate someone) requires even more engagement: in addition to focusing on what's being said, you need to fill in the blanks. Someone who's trying to organize their thoughts in real time is limited by any number of constraints (working memory capacity, anxiety, needing to pee, etc.). Attending has you mentally join the other person in trying to make their point. You consider how the information they're providing relates to other things you know about them or the world and try to develop an understanding that is more complete than what they're able to construct for you on the fly.

This type of engagement comes easily when you understand or at least care about the topic of discussion; it can be excruciatingly painful if you don't. Seeing clients from adolescents to older adults, I frequently find myself in conversations I'm not particularly interested in having. That's putting it mildly. Half the time, I don't understand what my clients are talking about. Can I believe that Jenna got doxxed on Discord? I guess I can't because I'm only loosely familiar with those terms. Isn't it bullshit that Erik is going up for promo after only being at a level five for less than a year? I've never met Erik and don't particularly care if he's going for "promo," much less appreciate what it means for him to be at a level five.

As a young therapist, I used to bite my nails mercilessly in these moments. The combination of anxiety over not understanding what my clients needed and sheer boredom meant I couldn't keep polish on my nails for more than a day. Fortunately, I found a workaround—or rather, I discovered a game I soon realized most good listeners were already playing.

The *A Game*,* as I call it, isn't complicated; you just have to answer this two-parter:

- What's a better way to make this person's point?
- Why does it matter to them?

Rules:

- Don't communicate your answers to the speaker. At least, not for the purposes of Attending. Like Sudoku or Solitaire, the A Game is one you play against yourself. It's technically possible to win without saying a word.
- You can ask the speaker questions and make comments, but you're limited to those that demonstrate *interest* or an effort to better *understand* their perspective. (See the "Ask Questions and Comment" section.)

To win the A Game, you must abandon the assumption that it's the other person's job to explain everything to you. Instead, it's up to you to figure out their message and why it matters to them. The challenge lies in finding a *better* way of framing the other person's point. This key element of the game is critical to overriding complacency and reining in your negativity bias. Our brains are quick to check one of the "I got it," "That's stupid," or "I don't care" boxes so we can go back to thinking about more important issues like, "What should I have for lunch?" or "Why *don't* they talk about Bruno?" If you accept the challenge of trying to flesh out someone's message, you move from passive judge to active participant.

Notice that nothing says you have to agree with or like the other person's perspective. Like a debate in which you're given a

---

* I call it the *A Game* because *A* is short for "Attending" and also because playing the *A Game* is how you bring your "A game" to your relationships. If you're thinking, "That's lame," then maybe my real intent was to give you an opportunity to practice cultivating that nonjudgment I'm always going on about. Only one of us will ever know for sure.

OBJECTIVE

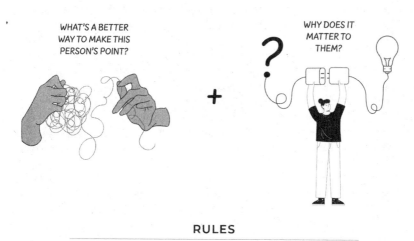

WHAT'S A BETTER
WAY TO MAKE THIS
PERSON'S POINT?

+

WHY DOES IT
MATTER TO
THEM?

?

RULES

· Do not share your answers with the speaker.

· Any questions or comments must demonstrate interest or an effort to understand the speaker's perspective.

random topic and need to argue a position, the A Game requires you to think in a way that engages you even if the subject matter doesn't. **The best validators all approach listening this way, not as the passive absorption of information but as the active construction of meaning.**

Ask Questions and Comment

If it's appropriate to talk to the other person while playing the A Game, you can, but you're limited to asking questions about their experience or commenting on it. Whether your questions and comments are perceived as Attending (or annoying) depends on *what* you ask and *how* you ask it.

For the purposes of Attending, your questions and comments **must demonstrate *interest* or an effort to *understand* someone better.** That's it. Statements like, "What do you think they meant by that?" "Were you surprised?" and "Wow," show interest, while

"Can you explain that to me?" and "Say that again" communicate an effort to understand.

The strongest Attending questions and comments reflect an interest in the other person *and* a desire to understand them. Although the prompt for DelGaudio's audience members was to pick a card, the task was a veiled way of asking, "How do you see yourself?" This question checks both the "Demonstrate interest" and "An effort to understand someone" boxes.

How you ask questions and make comments is as important as what you say. Enter, vocal cues. Consider the question, "Do you think you're a good father?" Try asking this question as judgmentally and critically as you can. Okay, now try asking the same question but in a gentle and supportive manner. Do you hear a difference? Asked one way, perhaps with a soft tone, a slow speed, and a slight inflection on "father," the question sounds thoughtful and curious. Said another way, with a sharp tone, a louder voice, and an emphasis on the "you," this same question feels like an attack.

If you've been accused of coming off as harsh despite not using language to that effect, you might be a victim of your vocal cues. I, for one, have always been a fast talker. Over the years, I've been forced to accept that this can sometimes come off as impatient or nervous. The trick to effectively managing quirks like talking quickly or robotically is to be aware of them. You don't have to fundamentally change your speech patterns, but if someone responds poorly to your attempts to engage, you should adjust your tone, speed, or volume.

If you're aware of your natural speech patterns, you can intentionally adjust them to create a validating effect. Because I'm a fast, animated talker, when I make a point to slow down, it's noticeable. Speaking slowly and methodically is a departure from my frenetic, ferret-like MO, and it signals to others that I'm being thoughtful and intentional. The opposite is true for someone like DelGaudio. He's clearly aware of his flat, monotone speaking style and becomes more animated when he wants to Attend and draw the audience's attention to certain emotions, like when he adjusted his tone to recognize the humorous nature of the person who identified herself as "a midnight toker." These shifts are subtle but no less impactful. **Anytime you change your natural speech patterns in response to someone, it shows that they've affected you. This means they have your attention.**

WHEN TO ATTEND

Attending is a matter of using the Big Four nonverbals, listening with intention by playing the A Game, and asking questions and making comments. You stand no chance of demonstrating understanding or empathy for someone if you haven't been paying attention to them, so you have to Attend on some level anytime you want to validate. The real question is, when do you *only* Attend? When do you rely on this skill alone rather than any of the others?

Sticking with Attending will serve you well when you don't understand or empathize with someone's position. If you find yourself stuck in a conversation at Thanksgiving with an uncle who won't shut up about his offensive political views, this is probably the only step you'll be able to take toward validating him. Attending is also the way to go any time talking would be inappropriate. When you want to validate without interrupting the other person—think meetings, funerals, parent-teacher conferences, etc.—Attending is your best friend.

EVEN YOUR BEST FRIEND CAN BETRAY YOU: ATTENDING MISTAKES AND SOLUTIONS

Using nonverbals, listening, and asking questions and making comments might seem foolproof, but these basic approaches can backfire. When Attending fails, it's usually because of intensity or timing.

Intensity

Eye contact can do a lot to communicate attentiveness and build connections. But in some scenarios, it will actually make it more difficult for others to open up to you. People tend to avoid eye contact when they're feeling embarrassed, guilty, ashamed, or, in some cases, sad. Asking questions in these scenarios can come off as invasive, causing people to shut down rather than open up. **If you bring too much intensity to a delicate moment, you risk crumbling it.** Intensity can be managed or corrected simply by reading the room. If someone seems ashamed, embarrassed, or insecure about a topic, dial back your questions and comments, don't force eye contact, tone down your vocal cues, and take a step back—literally.

Timing

People talk when they want to talk, not when *you* want them to talk. Try asking kids "How was your day?" when you pick them up from school, and you'll see what I mean. Demanding that people be vulnerable or expecting them to engage simply because you're ready to Attend to them rarely goes over well. Although our intentions might seem benevolent—we're trying to connect; what could be wrong with that?—we actually may be responding more to our own needs than attending to another's. We want to fill a silence that makes us uncomfortable, satisfy our curiosity, or prove that we're a good parent, friend, spouse, etc. Such motivations run counter to the spirit of validation, which is to focus, almost meditatively, on another person's experience. **Attending to someone who doesn't want your attention reflects a lack of awareness. It isn't validating; it's just annoying.**

There's nothing wrong with asking questions like, "How was work?" or "What happened at school?" as long as you don't expect too much in return or beat people over the head with follow-up questions like you're using a crowbar to pry into their life (e.g., "How was school?" "Just fine?" "Why aren't you talking more?" "Did something happen?" "What happened?!"). Instead, focus on demonstrating interest and curiosity to the unprompted statements that come when you least expect them. Spontaneous comments are like cracked doors signaling that the other person is ready to let you in. People rarely provide clear signals like, "Honey, I could really use some validation around my frustrations with this guy at work." Instead, they say, "My colleague, Alex, is such a pain in the ass," and they raise the topic in bed when you're about to fall asleep rather than at dinner when you asked, "How was your day?" I'm not saying you should forgo sleep or read into every side comment. I am simply saying that Attending to the discussions people initiate can offer more opportunities to deepen your relationship than trying to force a conversation.

If it seems like people rarely open up to you or if you're looking to rekindle a connection that's gone cold, be intentional about finding times that are conducive to intimate conversation. After dinner, coffee dates, walks, late-night texts, and car rides are perfect scenarios for deep convos. You can expect a low return on investment if you approach people immediately before or after work, school, or other demanding activities because folks are typically focused on preparing or recovering from them. When you do get the spark you're seeking, be careful not to blow on it too hard. Allow for silence, especially if it feels like the moment might slip through your fingers if you don't keep stoking it with questions. If the other person changes the subject, try only once to return to it. If they don't bite, let it go. People don't open up in response to being pushed; they just become less likely to seek you out in the future.

RECAP

- Attending means paying attention and listening without judgment in a way that shows interest and cultivates understanding.
- You can Attend by doing the following:
  » Using the Big Four nonverbal behaviors—eye contact, proximity, gesturing, and nodding.

» Listening with intention by playing the A Game:
1. What's a better way to make the other person's point?
2. Why does it matter to them?

» Asking questions and making comments. Stick to those that demonstrate *interest* or show that you're genuinely trying to *understand*.

- Attending is always necessary for validation. You should rely exclusively on this skill if you don't yet understand or empathize with another person's perspective or if it's inappropriate to speak.

- Attending mistakes include the following:

» Using too much intensity.
Solution: Read the room. Adjust accordingly.

» Trying to force opportunities to Attend, rather than leaning into them when they naturally arise.
Solution: Wait for people to open up, and don't flood them when they do.

PRACTICE TIPS

1. If you can commit the Big Four to memory and remember to lean into nonverbals in general, you should be good to go. You might put a reminder on your phone or fridge to cue you to be mindful of nonverbals this week, but don't overthink what you're doing in the moment.

2. A couple of the skills in the Validation Ladder are less intuitive and have aspects you need to drill to internalize. The A Game component of Attending is one of them. In my experience, playing the A Game usually starts to become second nature after about twenty-five repetitions. To develop your A Game, practice playing it in the following scenarios this week:

» Low-stakes conversations on issues you care about
(e.g., talking to your partner about the podcast you're
both listening to).

» Low-stakes conversations on topics that aren't of
interest to you (e.g., talking to your partner about the
Catan podcast they just finished).

» Low-level disagreements or conversations when you
don't understand someone's position (e.g., talking
with your partner about the *I Hate Cats* podcast
they've been enjoying).

Hint: Remember to ask questions and make comments that demonstrate interest or an effort to deepen your understanding. And nothing says these conversations need to happen live and in person. Electronic communication is still communication.

CHAPTER 7

COPY—HOW TO CONNECT
WITH ANYONE

I live in the facial expressions of the other, as I feel him living in mine.

—MAURICE MERLEAU-PONTY, *THE PRIMACY OF PERCEPTION*

Reader, I love this chapter. Partly because I get to talk about my husband talking about Seth Rogen talking about magic mushrooms, but also because I get to share my one-step plan for world peace. There's a lot to cover, so I'm going to jump right in.

Copying is the second of the two **Mindfulness Skills**, and it's as straightforward as they come: You simply mimic or reflect a person's words or behavior.* This skill is most effective when combined with Attending questions and comments. For example, someone says, "That restaurant was the best I've been to in years,"

---

* Reflect Back, Accurate Reflection, Mimicking, Mirroring, Speaker/Listener, Paraphrasing, and Reflective Listening are all variations of this same skill. (Linehan, *DBT Skills Training*, "Handout 18"; Linehan, "Validation and Psychotherapy," 362; Mariëlle Stel and Roos Vonk, "Mimicry in Social Interaction: Benefits for Mimickers, Mimickees, and Their Interaction," *British Journal of Psychology* 101, no. 2 [May 1, 2010]: 311–23, https://doi.org/10.1348/000712609x465424; Tom Bunn, "Megaphone Parenting Can't Meet a Child's Need for Mirroring," *Psychology Today*, September 16, 2019, https://www .psychologytoday.com/us/blog/conquer-fear-flying/201909/megaphone-parenting-cant-meet-childs-need-mirroring; Scott D. Stanley, Howard J. Markman, and Susan L. Blumberg, "The Speaker/Listener Technique," *The Family Journal* 5, no. 1 [January 1, 1997]: 82–83, https://doi.org/10.1177/1066480797051013; Kerry Patterson et al., *Crucial Conversations Tools for Talking When Stakes Are High*, 2nd ed. [New York: McGraw Hill Professional, 2011], 164; Alain Braillon and Françoise Taiebi, "Practicing 'Reflective Listening' Is a Mandatory Prerequisite for Empathy," *Patient Education and Counseling* 103, no. 9 [September 1, 2020]: 1866–67, https://doi.org/10.1016/j.pec.2020.03.024.)

while smiling. You respond, "The best in years?" matching their smile (Copying). "What did you order?" (Attending question). Some degree of summarizing and word swapping is fine, but Copying is most validating when it maps as directly onto what the person expressed as possible. I'll explain how to be effective, and not obnoxious, with this in a moment.

It might not seem like Copying a person could be validating, but, remember, as a **Mindfulness Skill**, it just needs to demonstrate that you're paying attention to someone without judging them. This might not seem like much, but, as we saw with Attending, acknowledging someone without judgment or bias can be incredibly moving. Derek DelGaudio's ability to create an experience in which "no one will feel judged" and "our 'I ams' become 'we are'" was largely achieved through Copying. He gave each person his undivided attention and said the words they felt best described themselves. He didn't offer any interpretations or elaborate on the descriptions people chose; he just repeated them verbatim.

Fortunately, you don't need to be a trained professional to reap the benefits of Copying. Research has shown that simply instructing someone to Copy another person positively affects how they feel about each other.[1] As you might expect by now, how people *feel* about each other affects how they *treat* one another. In perhaps the most famous study on Copying, researcher Rick B. van Baaren and his colleagues instructed waiters to either repeat or not repeat their patrons' orders.[2] They found that customers who'd had their orders repeated left significantly larger tips. Similar results were reported in a follow-up study on Copying and prosocial behavior.[3] In this experiment, researchers either Copied or did not Copy the leg and arm positions of participants during a one-on-one conversation. Participants were not aware they were being Copied. The conversation lasted only six minutes, after which the experimenter "accidentally" dropped some pens on the floor. Participants who had unknowingly been Copied by the experimenter picked up the pens more often (100 percent) than those who had not been Copied (33 percent).

And before you start daydreaming about all the tips you'll get and pens people will pick up for you, remember that Copying, like all validation skills, affects the validator as much as it does the person being validated. **Research has shown that the person Copied and the Copier *both* report more connection and a stronger emotional bond with each other.**[4] This is a really important point! Like, bust out a highlighter, text a friend, put it on a mug so you never forget it important. Because the more closely attuned and bonded we are to an individual, the harder it is for us to justify treating them poorly. If Copying someone really does cause us to feel more connected to them, then this one validation skill has the potential to reduce discrimination. In fact, it has proven to do just that.

In 2012, a group of non-Black participants was randomly subdivided into one of three groups. Students in the first group were instructed to watch a video of a Black actor and Copy his movements as he repeatedly reached for and drank from a cup of water. Those in the second group were told to watch the video *without Copying* the actor. The third group was given the same instructions as the first, except the actor they watched and Copied was *non-Black* like them. Participants then completed a task designed to measure implicit racism. Implicit racism refers to an unconscious prejudice that may cause a person to behave in a biased manner even though they do not intend to be discriminatory.[5] In the end, participants who Copied the Black actor showed an absence of implicit prejudice, while those in the other two groups showed an implicit bias against Black people. The researchers of this study suggest that the connection that results from Copying someone might cause us to see them less as an "other" and more like ourselves.[6]

If you're thinking, "Well, maybe the people randomly assigned to Copy the Black actor happened to harbor less implicit racism than those in the other group," then you might prefer an experiment that uses a pre-post design. In these studies, researchers measure participants' scores before (pre) and after (post) a task to see if the task affects their scores. Enter Xbox. In the most ingenious use of the Xbox 360 Kinect game *Dance Central 3* ever recorded, Ron Tamborini and colleagues at Michigan State University showed that white participants who closely Copied the dance moves of a Black virtual dancer for three songs rated Black people as significantly *more* trustworthy than they had before completing the task.[7] These effects were completely dependent on how synchronized the participants were with the virtual dancers: the better participants were at Copying the dancer's movements, the more pronounced the effects appeared to be.

These studies provide just a tiny glimpse into the effect Copying has on affiliation. Others show that Copying reduces victim-blaming,[8] compels people to give more to charity,[9] and increases their empathy toward citizens on opposite sides of a war.[10] In the realm of dating, Copying even has been shown to increase attraction.[11] The only way this skill could get any better is if it was easier to use. Just kidding; it's so easy a baby could do it. Literally.

MONKEY SAY, MONKEY DO

You've got two main options when it comes to using this skill to validate others: Copy their words and Copy their ways.

Copy Their Words

I wanted to provide as organic of an example as I could of Copying someone's exact words in a conversation, so I went undercover. One evening during dinner, I asked Mat to tell me about the book he was reading. Unbeknownst to him, I was making a point to Copy him and recording the conversation on my phone so I could transcribe it for you below. I told Mat afterward about my stealth operation, and he was cool with me including it in the book.

Okay, so he was reading Seth Rogen's autobiography *Yearbook*. Yes, this is when I get to talk about Mat talking about Rogen talking about shrooms. I'm sorry; I know you didn't sign up for a story about illicit drug use when you bought this book on validation, but here we are.

Mat: They were going to eat them [the shrooms], get their groceries, then go on a picnic. They figured the drugs would kick in when they got to the park. But, nope, it hit them like instantly when they were at the grocery store.

Me: Before they bought anything? [Attending question].

Mat: Yeah. [Mat starts laughing.] Seth ends up giving all his money to the cashier and leaving with the food. They finally get to a beautiful park in Amsterdam, but Seth has to poop, so he tells his friend, "I'm going to be right back. I just have to find a bathroom." And the guy's like, "Please, whatever you do, don't leave me right now!" The guy is like in tears.

Me: "Oh. He's crying?" [Attending question + Copying].

Mat: 'Cause he's so high. But Seth has to poop really badly so he's like, "I gotta go right now or things are gonna get very weird and bad."

We both laugh.

Me: They're in a beautiful park and he has to poop. [Copying].

More laughing.

Mat: So he finds a bathroom, and when he comes back, he sees his friend lying face down with his arms at his side, and Seth is very alarmed because the friend looks dead. So, he says, "Hey, what's going on?" and his friend says, "I'm hiding."

Me: "I'm hiding?!" [Copying].

We both crack up!

Mat: Yes! He's like, "I'm trying to stay perfectly still so no one sees me." Seth is like, "What are you talking about? No one is looking at you." And then his friend goes, "Then it's working."

Me: "Then it's working" [Copying]. That's hilarious.*

---

* I realize there's a lot of laughing going on. I just want to clarify that Mat and I were not on drugs. Although we do seem to have some sort of contact high because the bits we're laughing at don't seem that funny when I read them back. This story *is* funny if you listen to Rogen tell it in his audiobook; just not so much when you hear Mat explaining it to me. I've made the unedited recording of our conversation available on my website (drcarolinefleck.com) if you want a better sense of how Copying "sounds." But I warn you, it's not funny.

This is a condensed version of our longer conversation, and my use of Copying appears a bit more obvious here than it is in the full transcript. I point this out because Copying is most effective when it's least perceptible. The key to being validating and not robotic with this skill is to combine it with Attending questions and comments like I do in the beginning of our conversation when I ask if they left before buying anything.

Repeating the adjectives or exact descriptions people use can be particularly effective because these words are like the paint color they've chosen for a particular detail (e.g., "they're in a beautiful park"). Repeating them confirms that you see what the other person sees and are aware of what strikes them as important. Copying the tone and stylistic approach someone uses in their emails and texts is another subtle way to Copy and signal attunement. And be sure to pay close attention to people's use of exclamation points and emojis, because these convey the tone, intensity, and level of formality the individual is comfortable with.

Summarizing or repeating the main points of a person's argument also qualifies as using this skill, presuming you stick to what they said and not your *interpretation* of what they said. Copying reflects the other person's position; interpretations, on the other hand, can muddle it. Again, you don't have to *agree* with someone to restate their position. I seriously doubt DelGaudio agreed with the person who saw themselves as "a nobody." He was simply validating that this is how the individual saw themselves.

As calculated as Copying sounds, you don't have to focus on all these strategies when you're doing it. My only thoughts going into my conversation with Mat were (1) Copy, and (2) be sure Havana doesn't overhear us talking about drugs. Having now learned these techniques, you'll find that you naturally gravitate toward them when you practice Copying. Watching other people use this skill and experimenting with it yourself will reinforce what you've learned so that eventually, when you decide to secretly record yourself having a conversation with your husband about Seth

Rogen, you'll have an exemplary example of Copying to share with the world. Presuming he lets you.

Copy Their Ways

Since I was a kid, I've struggled with an issue I'm embarrassed to acknowledge. *Deep breath* . . . This is hard for me . . . I unknowingly Copy people's accents. I don't mean to, I really don't, but if I'm not careful, I'll start to adopt the accent of whomever I'm speaking with, often to a comical degree. If I've had a glass of wine, forget it. I'll be full-on talking like I'm from their country of origin.

I was relieved to learn that the tendency to Copy accents is common and not driven by an unconscious desire to mock people but rather by an unknowing attempt to validate them. Sometimes referred to as the chameleon effect, research confirms that we naturally Copy the accents, vocal tendencies, behaviors, and facial expressions of people we talk to.[12] In fact, we're hardwired to Copy how people speak and behave. Studies of babies show that they have a natural tendency to mimic facial and emotional expressions.[13]

Unconsciously Copying each other might seem like a weird tic for the human race to have developed, but, as with all hereditary traits, this one appears to have served an evolutionary function. To stay alive, you need a tribe. To build a tribe, you must be able to understand and empathize with people. Copying, it turns out, helps us do just that.[14]

Our brains associate certain facial expressions and muscular contractions with specific emotions. Drawing your eyebrows inward and downward, for example, is associated with anger. Stimulating these eyebrow muscles by Copying an angry facial expression can cause you to feel angry. Copying expressions associated with specific emotions activates the brain's motor cortex *and* regions used in processing emotions. By way of this trusty little feedback loop, Copying people helps us better understand and empathize with them.[15] Again, these effects are not one-directional. Copying leads *both* the Copier and the person being Copied to feel more closely connected, share similar emotions, and even report smoother interactions with each other.[16] Copying appears to be nature's way of helping you develop the capacity to more deeply empathize with others while simultaneously validating them in the process. Leave it to nature to be efficient as hell.

So whether or not you realize it, you already know that Copying people's words and ways is validating, and you're already doing it on some level to establish and maintain your tribe. I'm suggesting that you Copy with more frequency and intention when trying to validate someone (unless you get carried away with accents, in which case, stay away from alcohol). The reason I encourage more intentionality is because we're not indiscriminate in our mimicry. On the contrary, we're more likely to Copy people who are attractive[17] and in positions of power.[18] If these are the only people you ever need to validate, you're good. If not, you'll be happy to know that *intentionally* Copying people is no less effective when doing it spontaneously.[19] Both yield the delicious fruits of understanding and connection.

Because we're already hardwired to Copy each other, most people don't need to make much effort beyond reminding themselves to do it.* When I botched my initial attempt to validate the overwhelmed nanny I met in the park, I realized I needed to regain my footing with the **Mindfulness Skills**. At the time, I didn't think to myself, "She's crossing her arms, so *I'll* cross *my* arms," or

---

* I emphasize that *most* people won't need more than a gentle self-reminder to Copy others because some will need additional support to develop this skill. Spontaneous Copying is reduced in people who score low on trait empathy, such as people with autism spectrum conditions (ASC). Research has shown that intentionally Copying others' facial expressions can help those with ASC learn to accurately identify and process other people's emotions. (Chun-Ting Hsu, Thomas B. Sims, and Bhismadev Chakrabarti, "How Mimicry Influences the Neural Correlates of Reward: An FMRI Study," *Neuropsychologia* 116 [August 18, 2017]: 61–67, https://doi.org/10.1016/j.neuropsychologia.2017.08.018; Michael Lewis and Emily Dunn, "Instructions to Mimic Improve Facial Emotion Recognition in People with Sub-Clinical Autism Traits," *Quarterly Journal of Experimental Psychology* 70, no. 11 [November 1, 2017]: 2357–70, https://doi.org/10.1080/17470218.2016.1238950.)

"Aha, she cocked her right eyebrow! Let me do the same. Oh shoot, I've never been able to cock my right eyebrow." Instead, I just registered that I should make a point to Copy her. A gentle self-reminder is typically all that's needed to draw out this natural tendency.

There's one last way to Copy for the purposes of validation that falls somewhere in between repeating what the other person said and mimicking their actions, and that is to give words to their actions. For instance, if Mat said "The house looks nice," after I'd spent the day deep cleaning and organizing everything, I might appreciate the compliment, but I wouldn't feel particularly validated. If instead he said, "The house looks nice. Wow, did you clean the windows?! They're sparkling! And are those handmade labels in the pantry? That must have taken hours!" then I'd know that he was mindful of the time and effort I put in. Holding up a mirror to someone's experience is an obvious, but often overlooked, way to show that you see them.

COPYING: THE CONFLICT CURE

As a **Mindfulness Skill**, you'll find that Copying works well in the same scenarios that lend themselves to Attending. Copying's ability to foster trust and understanding also makes it an excellent antidote for conflict.

After conducting thousands of hours of research on relationships, John Gottman and his wife, psychologist Julie Gottman, developed an approach to couples therapy based on their prolific findings. Gottman Method Couples Therapy is one of a handful of proven treatments for couples hoping to improve or salvage their relationships. When I was first learning this therapy, I was expected to practice using the Gottmans' various methods with my clients. John Gottman is famously known as the dude who can predict if a couple will divorce, with more than 90 percent accuracy.[20] A randomized clinical study showed that partners who simply read his book *The Seven Principles for Making Marriage Work* were significantly happier in their relationship as far out as a year after reading it.[21] What therapist wouldn't want to put Gottman's methods into practice? That's what I thought until I encountered the Gottman-Rapoport Intervention (known simply as Rapoport).[22]

One of Gottman's key conflict management methods, Rapoport seemed so contrived I didn't see how I could use it without compromising my self-respect. My aversion might seem extreme, but consider what the intervention requires: As the therapist, I'd have to interrupt a couple's argument to suggest that one person abandon whatever point they are trying to make. Instead, I'd instruct them to listen to and repeat the other person's perspective, making adjustments until the speaker is satisfied with the listener's understanding. Because, you know, nothing brokers peace like forcing one side to represent the other's position through gritted teeth while being repeatedly told that they're getting it wrong. To make matters worse, I was supposed to hand the listener a clipboard so they could write down (Copy) what the speaker was saying. "Ladies and gentlemen, I interrupt your regularly scheduled fight to bring you a writing assignment," is what this sounded like to me. After the speaker is satisfied with the listener's summary, the two would switch places. I wasn't sure I'd be able to keep both partners in the room long enough for that to happen. I could only imagine the feedback I'd get from clients afterward: "Everything was going fine until she forced a really awkward exercise on me and my wife. The awkwardness has permanently stained our relationship, and we see no option now but to divorce. . . ."

As luck would have it, shortly after learning Rapoport, I did an escape room, which, if you haven't done one, is where you pay money to have yourself locked in a room with your friends to solve puzzles. We were given these adorable electronic notepads called Boogie Boards so we could write down clues and easily erase them after each puzzle. I love office gadgets and immediately realized that I could use the Boogie Board in lieu of clipboards for the notetaking part of Rapoport. If doing Gottman's intervention was the only way I could justify buying this toy, then so be it. Nothing stands between me and office supplies. I got me a couple of Boogie Boards and started experimenting with using Rapoport to help couples navigate conflicts in session. And let me tell you, it worked like magic! Probably because it is magic. I mean, it's basically the same "magic" DelGaudio was using.

The utility of the Rapoport exercise was evident to people almost immediately. Assuring the first listener that they'd get a chance to tell their side of the story was enough to overcome any initial resistance. Rather than being put off by the "writing assignment," most people are eager to show how well they've been listening, even if only to prove it to themselves.

So why is Copying such a potent antidote for conflict? Because the challenge of trying to repeat someone's points correctly forces you to slow way down. **When you downshift from the high gear of generating counterarguments and preparing critiques to processing and Copying, you see things you would otherwise miss.** It's the difference between speeding down the highway and slowly navigating a neighborhood. You have more time to process what's happening when you go slowly; it's easier to brake and avoid running over people. With Copying working in the background to foster understanding and empathy, important details come into focus, making it easier for you to see the "we are"s through the "I am"s.

Gottman said he developed the Rapoport intervention based on Anatol Rapoport's book *Fights, Games, and Debates*, which proposes strategies for international conflict resolution. Having seen what the Rapoport intervention is capable of, I have no doubt it would serve the global community well. Plus, how cute would it be to see world leaders reading off the notes they took on their Boogie Boards in their efforts to validate each other? Instant world peace! Okay, maybe not. But attempting to absorb another person's argument well enough to accurately repeat it will help you loosen some knots when you feel the tension tightening around a discussion. You don't necessarily have to write down what the other person is saying if you think it'll be awkward to do so, but if you experiment with this approach, you'll find few people take offense to you (literally) noting their concerns.

COPYING MISTAKES

Because we come by Copying naturally, this skill isn't as fraught with potential mistakes as some of the others. You'll have problems with Copying only if you fail to balance it with Attending or draw attention to what you're doing. Some therapists encourage people to use preambles like "I hear you saying . . ." as a lead-in to Copying someone's words. I disagree. In my experience, these types of statements can come across as phony or even judgmental. Better to focus on Copying, not make a production of it. This "don't make a production of it" advice might seem contradictory coming from the woman advocating for note-taking during arguments. But in the latter situation, the aim is to help you do a better job of Copying, not to draw attention to yourself. The props are quickly forgiven once they've fulfilled their function.

Relying on a gentle self-reminder to Copy, rather than obsessively monitoring yourself, will help you draw out your natural tendency to Copy without being obvious or forcing it. The only other thing to be mindful of is which behaviors you Copy. Never, ever Copy someone who is being aggressive, rude, or violent. Copying nonverbal expressions of sadness or distress (e.g., looking down, tearing up, etc.) can be validating; you just want to be careful not to cross the line into overwhelming someone. **Copying ceases to be effective the minute the situation feels like it's spiraling out of control.** Signs of spiraling include looks of panic, distress, and uncontrollable sobbing. When this happens, stop Copying and start soothing.

Copying young children can give you a real feel for what it's like to cross the line from comfort to chaos and back again. Kids benefit greatly from the validation they experience in seeing their emotions reflected by an adult. It shows them that their feelings are real, are appropriate to the situation, and can be trusted. Kids are also notoriously poor at emotion regulation, which makes Copying their negative emotions a bit like walking on a tightrope. Earlier this week, for example, Havana called me back into her room after I'd put her to bed, saying she was worried she might have a nightmare. "Nightmares are so scary, I'd rather not sleep at all!" she said with wide eyes. "Some *are* really scary," I said, repeating her adjective and widening my eyes. Reader, this was not the right move! She burst into tears as if I'd literally confirmed her worst nightmare. I quickly switched gears and scooped her up in my arms. "But remember," I said, "we can think loving thoughts to help keep nightmares away! I'll go first . . ." That last bit of advice is only loosely based on science, and yes, I sometimes exaggerate effects to help my kid fall asleep. The point is that the transition from validating to soothing doesn't have to be graceful; it just needs to happen.

RECAP

- Copying means mirroring someone's words (what they say) or ways (gestures and expressions) or putting words to their ways (acknowledging their efforts).
- Copying works in any situation that warrants Attending. It is also particularly helpful during conflicts.
- When Copying, be careful not to:
  » Make a big deal out of it.
    Solution: Balance Copying with Attending questions and comments, and gently remind yourself to Copy without excessive self-monitoring.
  » Copy the wrong behavior.
    Solution: Never Copy aggressive behavior; if you go overboard with Copying negative feelings like sadness, stop Copying and start soothing.

PRACTICE TIPS

1. Use the prompt "Remember to Copy" to cue yourself to intentionally Copy someone each day this week. Put a virtual sticky note on your computer or an actual one on your mirror to remind yourself to do it.

2. The next time you find yourself in conflict, try the Rapoport intervention. You can do it formally by writing down what the other person says or informally by trying to keep track of their points in your head. If the person is an intimate partner or family member, you might try introducing the exercise to them so you both have the opportunity to be heard.

CHAPTER 8

CONTEXTUALIZE— SOLVING FOR WHY

I myself have always found that if I examine something, it's less scary.
—JOAN DIDION, *THE CENTER WILL NOT HOLD*

When my friend Kim's son, Jeff, entered first grade, he was possessed by an evil demon. At least, that's how it seemed to us. Gone was the sweet child who'd once asked if he could bring ants inside to keep them safe from the rain. In his place was a boy bent on destruction and disruption. Kim was first called to the school in September, when Jeff was caught drawing on his desk with a Sharpie he'd stolen from home; phone calls from the school soon became a weekly thing. As the year dragged on, his teacher's patience grew thin. Kim asked to speak with her after Jeff claimed she called him a jerk. "I said he was *acting* like a jerk, not that he *is* a jerk," the teacher clarified. Kim was pissed.

Jeff's teacher ended up leaving the school in January. Kim held out hope that things might be better with the new teacher. And they were, for all of one day; then Jeff started having trouble again. Kim wasn't surprised when she got a message from the new teacher requesting a meeting. She was, however, surprised by the teacher's approach: rather than digging into Jeff's behavior, she focused on gathering information. Did he have issues in kindergarten? Any problems with friends? "Wait, what's that?" she asked when Kim mentioned that Jeff refused to practice reading at home and had a meltdown whenever he had to work on assignments outside of school. "Hmm," she mused.

A few weeks later, the teacher referred Jeff to a learning specialist, who ran a battery of tests over several days. "He has dyslexia," Kim told me after meeting with the school to discuss the results. "I feel so bad!" Jeff wasn't a problem child; he was struggling. His teacher immediately stopped sending his unfinished classwork home for him to complete and began meeting with him after school to review lessons and lavish him with praise while he sat on a throne (aka the teacher's chair). With the punishment and reinforcement balances tipped in reinforcement's favor, the demon stood no chance. By the end of the year, Jeff was back to the gentle child we'd always known him to be.

None of us could understand Jeff's behavior at the beginning of the year. It was outside the norm and ran counter to the classroom culture. It was also wildly ineffective: he was always in trouble and seemed angry much of the time. After we learned about his dyslexia, though, Jeff's behavior made more sense. This additional information was enough to transform everyone's understanding and enable them to validate him. Herein lies the power of Contextualizing.

Although Jeff's reaction to first grade wasn't "normal," it was understandable in the context of his learning disorder and the fact that he was struggling to keep up. **Contextualizing acknowledges that a person's reaction makes sense in some context—their physiology, history, etc.—even if it's problematic or ineffective otherwise.*** In these situations, validation is based on the assumption that every effect has a cause.

To Contextualize, you must first determine the chain of cause and effect that led to someone's reaction and then communicate it.

---

* Contextualizing is also known as Communicate an Understanding of the Causes, Historicizing, and Validating in Terms of Sufficient (but Not Necessarily Valid) Causes. (Linehan, *DBT Skills Training*, "Handout 18"; Linehan, "Validation and Psychotherapy," 367.)

The chain doesn't need to be elaborate. Here are some examples I gathered during the past week to give you a sense of what I mean:

I'll stay up here with you. There's no snakes down there, but I know you're scared there might be because of when you were little.

—Havana, Contextualizing the irrational fear of snakes her grandma
developed after boys put garden snakes down her dress as a kid

My talk is about depression, and I am currently in a depression right now, and if you are familiar with it, then you're probably familiar with that exhausted brain fog that makes you unable to remember anything at all, which is the reason why I have brought my notes out with me. It's ugly, but honestly, so is depression sometimes, so fuck it.

—Jenny Lawson, Contextualizing her "exhausted brain fog" and use of
notes during a TEDx Talk[1] (Hurray for self-validation!)

I totally get it. With MS, you've got to be extra careful about protecting your health.

—An administrator Contextualizing my request to teach
remotely post-lockdown even though the department
required us to return to in-person instruction

The trick to Contextualizing isn't figuring out what to say. As you can see from my examples, the message is always some variation of "given x, y makes sense." It's more about finding the connection between x and y. Like the other **Understanding Skills** in this chapter, Contextualizing is based on logical reasoning. It requires deduction first and communication second. The moment you shift from judging someone's reaction—our default, thanks to the negativity-bias devil—to solving for it, you increase your chances of being able to validate them. Contextualizing facilitates understanding by disarming two of its greatest foes: shoulds and fear.

SHOULDS

Have you heard the expression, "Stop shoulding all over yourself?" If not, say it out loud (unless your kids are around). The point is that we hold ourselves to unrealistic expectations and then get all hot and bothered when we fail to meet them. But we don't just save the judgments for ourselves; we should all over others, too. And the more we focus on how someone "should be," the harder it is to accept them as they are.

Contextualizing is one way to put an end to the should show:

"My son is twelve years old; he should be able to get his homework done without me constantly having to remind him!" *No, he shouldn't! You've been reminding him to do his homework since he was first assigned any. He hasn't developed the skills to task-manage independently, and your reminders have saved him from ever having to deal with the natural consequences of missing assignments.*

"I should have stopped reminding him years ago." *No, you shouldn't have! You didn't realize reminders could be contributing to the problem until just now when I mentioned it. In theory, you could have had different information and resources and lived a different life, but you didn't. You lived the life you're living. And in the context of that life, your parenting decisions make sense.* **There's a valid reason you're doing the things you're doing, and it's not that you suck.**

The key to Contextualizing, and to challenging shoulds in general, is to remember that *understanding ≠ approval*. It's not the same as condoning someone's behavior, and there's nothing to say that by accepting the current conditions, you sacrifice your ability to change them in the future. Explanations are not excuses. The teacher who tries to understand the factors contributing to a child's disruptive behavior is more likely to succeed in changing it than the one who writes him off as a jerk.

FEAR

It is incredibly difficult to connect with those we feel the need to protect against. A first-grader can start to seem like a "bad guy" if he consistently threatens the peace you're trying to keep. As I discussed in chapter 2, negative emotions like fear and its first cousin, anger, can activate our fight/flight/freeze response, undermining our ability to reason. Even if our nervous systems haven't jumped off the sympathetic arousal cliff, emotions can still compromise our objectivity: the more frustrated Jeff's original teacher felt, the more judgmental she became.

But we don't have to remain trapped in the fun-house mirrors of our negative emotions. **Although it's true that feelings affect our reasoning, it's also true that reasoning affects how we feel.** Determining validity requires an unbiased assessment of someone's response. This thoughtful analysis leads to understanding, which is a catalyst for empathy and compassion. Recall that the **Empathy Skills** at the top of the Validation Ladder depend on understanding and will fail without it. In the context of validation, the mind is a conduit to the heart.

In addition to inspiring empathy and compassion, Contextualizing reduces those fiery emotions that distance us from others and distort reality. As the late Joan Didion observed, "if I examine something, it's less scary."[2] Once we see that we don't need protection, it becomes that much easier to establish a connection. Contextualizing and the other **Understanding Skills** help us realize that most of the monstrous shadows we encounter are nothing more than small hands in front of a flashlight.

This is usually about the point in my Contextualizing spiel when someone in the back row yells out, "But what about the monsters?" Or a person in the front row politely raises a hand and asks some version of "How do you validate someone who behaved immorally or committed a crime, and why would you want to?"

These are good questions because nowhere is Contextualizing more difficult than when understanding feels dangerous.

If the "monster" is someone in a position to physically, sexually, financially, or emotionally abuse you or those in your care, then fear is justified and you should follow your instinct to seek protection. Someone who is being abused is not in a position to change their abuser's behavior. Validation won't work in an abusive dynamic because contingencies cannot be enforced. The only person a victim of abuse should validate is themselves by leaving the situation at the first opportunity.

If the person in question is *not* someone you need protection from, your instincts can backfire. Fear gives us tunnel vision. It narrows our attention to what's wrong to the exclusion of everything else. The result is that we tend to reduce the "criminal" to their crime. They did something bad; therefore, they are bad and need to be punished. If we don't shame and invalidate them, they'll just keep doing what they're doing, or so fear tells us.

But fear is a liar. The last thing people need is more shame and invalidation. Most of the time, when someone behaves poorly, they feel bad about it. If they are lucky, their hurt will be contained to feelings of guilt. Guilt says, "I did bad." When hurt is compounded by negative feedback from others or internalized as a character flaw, it galvanizes into shame. Shame says, "I am bad." Here's where the trouble lies. People who think they've done something wrong can apologize and work on changing their behavior. People who believe they are bad are left with few options.

Fear tells us that rubbing people's noses in their mistakes will prevent them from acting out again, but nose rubbing only makes them more dangerous. People are not pacified by shame; they respond violently to it. Shame is highly correlated with self-destructive behaviors like self-harm, eating disorders, suicidal ideation, etc.,[3] and externalizing behaviors such as domestic violence, violent offenses, and bullying.[4] It also appears to play a causal role in the development of personality traits like narcissism and even psychopathy.[5] In the words of Karl Marx, "Shame is a kind of anger turned in on itself. And if a whole nation were to feel ashamed it would be like a lion recoiling in order to spring."[6]

You don't encourage good behavior by convincing someone they're bad. Instead, you must affirm that they're a decent person who made a mistake. You may need to set contingencies and enforce consequences along the way, but this must be done alongside understanding, not in place of it. Identifying the valid reasons why someone did the destructive things they did helps them understand their reaction and ways to avoid it in the future. If shame is the strange city they find themselves lost in, Contextualizing is the map that shows them how they got there—and how to get back out.

FINDING THE VALIDITY IN PROBLEM BEHAVIOR

Behavior doesn't occur in isolation; it occurs in context. **So in order to validate behavior that doesn't make sense, you must find the context in which it does.** In 1997, Marsha Linehan wrote a chapter on validation in a book about psychotherapy and identified three contexts in which problematic behavior may be valid: (1) the past, (2) misinformation, and (3) disorder.[7] The chapter is targeted to therapists but applies to anyone with a pulse because, like death, taxes, and poor Wi-Fi signals, problematic behavior is unavoidable. The contexts Linehan identified aren't the only ones in which problematic behavior may be valid, but they are some of the most common.

The Past
Conditioning is the fancy term behavioral scientists use to describe how associations made in the past affect current behavior. I should note that associations made during childhood and trauma often persist well after the circumstances have changed. A man who grew up in a home where yelling was consistently paired with physical violence might feel distressed and start to shut down when his wife raises her voice during a fight. If his wife comes from a fiery family in which heated arguments were associated with resolution, she would understandably feel frustrated and

push to reengage her partner when he shuts down. Each person's reaction is valid in terms of their *conditioning,* even if it's not effective in the moment.

Associations made in the context of intense pleasure and pain also get ironed in pretty well. Many folks who struggled with addiction show a spike in dopamine and an increased desire to use when encountering drug paraphernalia, even after being sober for years.[8] Meanwhile, ever since getting third-degree burns from his shirt catching the flames of our gas stove, Mat keeps an exaggerated distance from stovetops when passing them, even if they're electric . . . or turned off.

I'm not suggesting that you should go around speculating about people's histories or constructing stories about their past to make sense of their behavior. Assuming that someone's relationship problems stem from "mommy/daddy issues" isn't validating; it's condescending.

If, however, there's an obvious connection between what you see in the present and what you know about someone's past, then acknowledging it can have a profound effect. Validating someone's behavior in the context of their history substantiates the acceptance you aim to convey. It says, "I see how the world has shaped you, and I don't judge you for it."

Misinformation

If you're not aware of anything in a person's past that would help explain their reaction in the present, you may still be able to Contextualize some part of it. As I discussed in chapter 3, someone's reaction might be a valid response to invalid thoughts. And what's the greatest source of invalid thoughts? Misinformation.

Not showing up for a dental appointment on Tuesday when your appointment card says you're scheduled for Thursday is valid. Whoever filled out your card made a mistake, but your behavior makes sense based on the misinformation you were given. The consequences of misinformation obviously can be more devastating than a missed dentist appointment. The bigger the consequence, the harder it is to Contextualize someone's behavior in terms of the misinformation driving it. Even when it's clear that someone is reacting to lies or propaganda, we're no less quick to judge them. How could they be so "gullible," or "stupid," or "ignorant"?! *Sigh.* These judgments are destroying us. They're dividing us. They compromise the respect that's needed for constructive dialogue; in the absence of that dialogue, we become more righteous, isolated, and hateful.

Martin Luther King Jr. said: "Like an unchecked cancer, hate corrodes the personality and eats away its vital unity. Hate destroys a man's sense of values and his objectivity."[9] Judgment gives rise to hate. It enables us to see others as less than: less intelligent, less moral, less human. Although objectivity is poisoned by judgments, hate cannot exist without them. **When you are Contextualizing behavior in terms of misinformation, it's not enough to identify the logical connection between the two. You must refrain from judging the person who was misled.**

Disorder

In addition to the past and misinformation, problematic behavior may be valid in terms of the biological dysfunction that's driving it. If your brain is depleted of serotonin, you will feel and act depressed. If it's flooded with dopamine, you'll find it difficult to sleep.[10] Even if someone's behavior conflicts with their goals, it may still be valid in the context of an existing physical or mental health disorder.

By and large, we're not a society that excels in discussing disorders, much less validating the spiderweb of ways in which they can affect a person. One of the most common concerns people have about Contextualizing in these circumstances is that they'll end up reinforcing behaviors that, despite being driven by disease, are still problematic: for example, "I know Mom's arthritis makes it hard for her to exercise, but validating the struggle will only make her less likely to try."

The inadvertent reinforcement concern can be put to rest by

reminding yourself that you need only *validate the valid*. For example, I can validate why someone dealing with pain from arthritis would stop exercising. "Your body is literally telling you to take it easy," I might say. Or "Our species would not have evolved very far if we responded to broken ankles by running on them." I can acknowledge that avoiding exercise is a valid reaction to physical pain *and* work with the person suffering from it to find ways of increasing exercise given their goals of staving off disease progression, reducing pain, and combating fatigue. Their resistance is valid given their disorder, but not their goals.

In my work, I'm constantly balancing the scales of Contextualizing a person's behavior in terms of their disorder and challenging them to change that behavior to achieve their goals. It makes total sense that someone with depression would spend the whole weekend in bed, ignoring text messages from friends and getting up only to use the bathroom. Depression will do that to a person. I can validate that their behavior is understandable in light of their condition. Doing so doesn't undermine my ability to assert that giving in to their depression will only make things worse. On the contrary, I need them to accept how their disorder affects them in order to motivate change.

Just as you don't want to jump to conclusions about people's pasts, you shouldn't assume someone has a disease just because you don't like or understand their behavior. Suggesting that a person's behavior is pathological because it's different is a surefire way to invalidate them. Difference ≠ disorder.*

RECAP

- Contextualizing acknowledges that a person's reaction makes sense in some context, even if it's problematic or ineffective otherwise.

---

* Actual disorder impairs a person's ability to work or function. If someone's behavior (excessive sleep, drug use, fear of public speaking, etc.) is interfering with their ability to complete daily activities, then you might consider referring them to a doctor.

- Contextualizing is based on logical reasoning. It's a way of saying, "Given x (context), y (reaction) makes sense." The trick is in solving for x.
- Contextualizing facilitates understanding by disarming two of its greatest foes: shoulds and fear.
  » Too much shame drives people to violence; enough understanding can lead them to change.
- If you're struggling to find the validity in problematic behavior, consider if it can be Contextualized in terms of the following:
  1. The past
     › A reaction that's problematic now may have been effective once upon a time.
     Warning: Hold your assumptions lightly.
  2. Misinformation
     › Behavior may be valid if it's based on invalid information.
     Warning: Don't judge people for believing the lies people tell them.
  3. Disorder
     › Dysfunctional behavior may be valid in terms of a person's disorder, even if it conflicts wildly with their goals.
     Warning: Difference ≠ disorder.

PRACTICE TIPS

1. We tend to respond to problematic behavior with shoulds and judgments, so use these thoughts as cues to Contextualize this week. If everyone around you happens to be especially well behaved, imagine how you might Contextualize to validate obnoxious behavior you read about or see in the media. Think about what you could say to communicate your "given x, y makes sense" logic, and take special note of any judgments that pop up in the process

(e.g., "I'm making excuses for them" or "They don't deserve it").

2. It's most critical and difficult to practice Contextualizing when someone's behavior is immoral or conflicts with your values, but you might not find yourself in these situations on a daily basis. To get some reps in this week, defer to the news or social media for examples of egregious behavior. If you don't have the information you need to figure out the conditions that led to someone's reaction, use what you know to draw some hypotheses about the circumstances that are most likely to have led them to do what they did.

Note: These are hypotheses you're drawing, not assumptions. Hypotheses are held lightly, can be disproven, and are nonjudgmental; assumptions presume truth in the absence of proof. Generating hypotheses is how we come to understand the world; making assumptions is the surest way to distort it.

CHAPTER 9

EQUALIZE—THE "ANYONE IN YOUR SHOES WOULD DO THE SAME" SKILL

When you see yourself in others, it is impossible to hurt anyone else.
—UNKNOWN

In the spring of 2020, I was found guilty of invalidating Havana by a jury consisting of me, Mat—later found to be an accessory to the crime—and Havana. We were unanimous in our decision: Mommy (and to a lesser extent, Daddy) effed up. Here's what happened: The three of us decided to go for a hike about forty-five minutes from our house. Havana started feeling carsick early in the drive, which meant that she was in suboptimal form by the time we arrived at the trail. At first, just her tummy was upset; having mothered her for seven years, though, I knew there was a good chance her mood would follow suit. She's always been quick to recover from car sickness physically, so I thought if I kept her distracted, maybe I could turn things around before we got off on the wrong foot. Yeah, right.

"OOOOOOWWWWW," she cried out in front of me after walking into a branch. We were less than ten minutes into our hike. Her scream drowned out the "I'm psyched to hike" rap I was singing (and writing on the fly) behind her. I testified before the court that I was, in fact, annoyed to have my rap disrupted by such an unnecessary proclamation of pain. Standing behind her, I saw that the branch had merely brushed her back and torso.

"That branch attacked me," she declared when I asked if she was okay.

"Are you still feeling sick?" I asked.

She glared at me as if to say, "Don't you dare suggest that I'm overreacting."

"No, I'm not pukey anymore. That tree just stabbed me in the back."

I inspected the thin branch. It didn't have any burs or thorns and looked about as threatening as a strand of pasta. I rolled up her shirt to where she said it hurt but found no scratches or skin irritation to substantiate her claims. "Let's keep going," I said, allowing some frustration to seep into my tone.

"Why don't you care that I was attacked?!" Havana demanded.

"I do care, babe, but you can't scream like that in the woods," I said. "Another hiker might think you're in danger."

"I am in danger! A branch attacked me!"

"Let's keep going," I said with more firmness and frustration.

Of course, it was only downhill from there. Highlights from the hike include Havana insisting that we sit down every ten minutes so she could rest her back, me and Mat lecturing her on the perils of being dramatic, and Havana suggesting we go back and cut down the branch to keep it from "attacking" anyone else.

Everyone was relieved to get home, especially Havana, who said she needed to shower but was in too much pain from the branch attack to lift her arms.

"I thought you said it hurt your back," I said, helping her out of her shirt.

"It did, but now moving my arm hurts, too . . ." and that's when I saw it. A tick deeply embedded in Havana's right shoulder blade. The surrounding tissue was red and swollen. I also should mention that this was the exact moment when I recalled the "Beware of Ticks" sign at the entrance to the park. Oops. Back on the trail, she could reach only as high as her lower back when I asked her to show me where it hurt. Not seeing anything, I relied on my assumptions—she's crabby from the car ride, she doesn't appreciate my mad rapping skills, etc.—to make sense of her reaction and, in my opinion, none of it justified her response. Of course, hindsight is 20/20, and if I knew then what I know now, I would have validated that her reaction was proportionate to the offense, and that I'd want to take it easy, too, if a tick was hanging a "Home Sweet Home" sign on my back. Simply put, I would have Equalized.

Equalizing communicates that a person's response is reasonable or justified in terms of the current situation and normal biological functioning.* It's the "anyone in your shoes would do the same" skill. Havana wasn't operating off of prior conditioning, health anxiety, or misinformation (although I clearly was). Her reaction was typical of a kid who'd been bitten by an tick.

Equalizing isn't more or less powerful than Contextualizing; they're just intended for different scenarios. For instance, if someone literally threw out a baby with the bathwater, you'd need to rely on Contextualizing, because their behavior is not equivalent to what most people do after bathing a child, and also, "What the hell?" If instead they said they're exhausted because they were up all night with their baby, who got a rash from some bathwater, then you could Equalize, because who wouldn't be tired after a sleepless night with a baby?

When someone's response is reasonable given the circumstances, rationalizing it in terms of some other context can be royally *in*validating. Consider the example of a parent who panics and speeds to the ER after hearing their son took a ball to the head during baseball practice. Contextualizing this parent's reaction in terms of the severe anxiety disorder they also suffer from, "It makes sense that you rushed to the ER given how anxious you

---

* Also known as Acknowledging the Valid, Validating as Reasonable in the Moment, and Normalizing. (Linehan, *DBT Skills Training*, "Handout 18"; Linehan, "Validation and Psychotherapy," 370; Alan E. Fruzzetti and Kate M. Iverson, "Mindfulness, Acceptance, Validation, and 'Individual' Psychopathology in Couples," in *Mindfulness and Acceptance: Expanding the Cognitive-Behavioral Tradition*, eds. Steven C. Hayes, Victoria M. Follette, and Marsha M. Linehan [New York: Guilford Press, 2004], 185.)

always are" would be all sorts of rude. Instead, acknowledging that the parent's response is what you'd expect from someone in their situation—"I'd have totally lost it if I were you"—confirms its inherent validity.

HOW TO EQUALIZE

Like the other **Understanding Skills**, Equalizing comes down to logical reasoning and communication.

Logical Reasoning

To determine if someone is acting normally, you have to compare their behavior against something. The default, relatively mindless approach is to see if their reaction is consistent with all of the info you've collected during your years observing human behavior:

> **Default Approach**
> Person's reaction = how people typically respond

Recognizing that it's common for people to cry after losing a loved one, for instance, doesn't seem to take any mental energy. You just know their reaction is normal; you don't have to think about it. There's nothing wrong with relying on autopilot deductions, but to reach this skill's full validation potential, you need to get comfortable using the Golden Rule approach, during which you imagine yourself in the other person's situation to see if their reaction squares with yours:

> **Golden Rule Approach**
> Person's reaction = how I'd respond

Consider the distinction between registering that a person's grief is understandable (default approach) and imagining how you would feel, what you would think, and what you would do after losing a loved one (Golden Rule approach). Big difference. Putting yourself in someone else's shoes, even if it's just through imagination, requires a higher level of cognitive processing that engages the brain's visual, motor, and sensory systems. Research suggests that the practice of actively imagining another person's experience allows us to better intuit their thoughts, feelings, and needs.[1] This means that the Golden Rule approach you use to Equalize can actually help generate empathy.

In law, the so-called Golden Rule approach, known as the Golden Rule argument,[2] is considered such a powerful catalyst for empathy that it's deemed improper in some states for lawyers to ask jurors to imagine themselves in the victim's position. The concern is that any strong emotions evoked by the Golden Rule approach could affect jurors' verdicts. Of course, combining logic with emotion is what validation is all about.

Communication

Sometimes I torture myself by thinking about the validating things I could have said to my daughter over the years if only I'd been more intentional. Instead of "Things don't always go how we expect them to," I imagine myself saying, "I'd be disappointed, too, if my friend canceled on me at the last minute." Instead of "It's okay that you didn't finish your draft by the last day; it's just a writing camp," I say, "I always feel crushed when I don't meet my goals." Instead of, "A mask-less Darth Vader is not going to sneak through your window and smother your face with his; he's not even real, now go to bed," I say, "I, too, was freaked out when Darth Vader took off his helmet the first time I saw *Return of the Jedi*. I should have known better than to let you get your first visual of old man Anakin before bed."

In my mental validation do-overs with Havana, I Equalize by saying that I'd react similarly if I were in her shoes. When she becomes a teenager, I'll probably have to come at this from a different angle. Right now, at age eight, she idolizes me. Hearing that I—a grown, capable, all-knowing adult—would have the same reaction she's having means her response is legit. But by the time she's seventeen, some of my shine will have worn off. There might be occasions when comparing myself to her is validating, but I'll most likely need to rely on better reference points. Saying, "I imagine any one of your friends would have done the same," when she describes leaving a party after someone spilled a drink on her, is more likely to resonate than, "I [your old, out-of-touch mom] would have left a party if someone spilled a drink on me."

Generally speaking, Equalizing in the first person—saying that someone's reaction is equal to how *you* would react—is the way to go if you're an authority figure or someone they look up to. Consider how deliciously validating it feels when a doctor puts themselves in your shoes by saying something like, "I would want a second opinion, too, if I were you," or "If it were my kid, I'd do the same." Yummy.

The third-person comparison—stating that someone's response is equal to how others would respond—may be more appropriate if you don't know the person or their situation well. When I complain to my bachelor brother about how difficult it's been to manage childcare this summer, and he says, "Yeah, all my friends with kids have been saying the shortage of camps this year is killing them," I feel more validated than if he were to say, "Yeah, if I had a kid, I'm sure I'd be frustrated by the lack of options, too."

Regardless of whether you're comparing their behavior to yours or someone else's, there's a trick you can use to help punch up the power of Equalizing, and that is to incorporate the Caroline Qualifier. Named by yours truly, after yours truly, the Caroline Qualifier sweetens the standard Equalizing message of "anyone in your shoes would react similarly" with some version of "and you're handling it better than most." I don't know if it's because I'm sensitive or have a skewed sense of "normal" after treating mental health disorders for so long, but I'm often struck by how "above average" people's reactions seem to me. When I put myself in their shoes or compare their response to my internal database of typical reactions, their response strikes me as above average.

When my colleague's surrogate had a miscarriage in her second term, she asked for time to discuss it during our weekly clinical consultation team. She said she was working against the urge to minimize and avoid her emotions; instead, she wanted to "feel her feels" and began attending a grief counseling group for support. The awareness, intention, and grace she brought to this experience were inspiring to witness. Despite being a therapist, I had no idea there were grief counseling groups for miscarriages, much less knew anyone who'd attended one. My colleague's grief seemed understandable and normal, but how she managed her emotions struck me as exceptional. I could authentically say that I'd be devastated and find it hard to work, too, if I were in her shoes. But from a validation perspective, it seemed equally important to add that I thought she was managing it better than I (and most others) would.

WHEN EQUALIZING IS CRITICAL

You can rely on the default or Golden Rule approaches to help you logically understand and begin to empathize with someone's experience. Depending on the relationship, it may be more effective to communicate your understanding in the first or the third person. **However you go about it, if someone has been invalidated for having a normal reaction to abnormal circumstances, Equalizing can have a significant effect.** That's putting it mildly. Being made to feel crazy is like being on a plane that's losing cabin pressure. In these situations, Equalizing is the oxygen mask people need to keep their wits about them.

When a Normal Reaction to an Abnormal Situation Has Been Invalidated

"Someone must have been telling lies about Josef K., for without having done anything wrong, he was arrested one fine morning."[3] This is the first line of Franz Kafka's *The Trial*, the story of a man who is apprehended at his home without ever being told why. Throughout the book, Josef K. is subjected to a maddening amount of bureaucratic bullshit as he awaits his "trial"—he can meet with a supervising official only if he wears a specific black coat, he's chastised for being late to a summons despite not having been told when to arrive, and he cannot get any information on his case or the charges. None of it makes any sense. When Josef K. becomes angry or attempts to take reasonable actions, he's ridiculed for being irrational. In this nonsensical reality, his normal reactions are constantly being invalidated.

What I love about *The Trial* is that despite the fact that it is unrealistic, there's something deeply familiar about Josef K.'s experience. Maybe it was a bizarre job you had where everyone seemed robotically happy despite working under crappy conditions or a gaslighting dynamic with someone who caused you to doubt your perceptions. Even something as mundane as being told you can't return a pair of jeans when you're within the return window can hit that Josef K. chord within us. But the more serious and all-consuming someone's version of *The Trial* is, the more vital it becomes to Equalize their reaction. To give you a sense of what I mean, I now turn to Marie Adler's story. *Content warning: rape and sexual assault are referenced in this example. You can go to the next section, "When the Abnormal Situation Is Perfectionism," to skip it.*

In 2016, the article "An Unbelievable Story of Rape"[4] won the Pulitzer Prize[5] for its bone-chilling exposé of Marie Adler, who, on August 11, 2008, claimed she was raped by a stranger while alone in her apartment. The article explains that Marie called 911 immediately after the assault. She was taken to a hospital, where she was described as being in "no acute distress." Her foster mother was concerned by the inconsistencies in how Marie presented; law enforcement was concerned about inconsistencies in her story and the details she kept remembering after the fact. Several days later, when investigators called Marie in for yet another round of questioning, she withdrew her statement and wrote a new one, saying: "I have had a lot of stressful things going on and I wanted to hang out with someone and no one was able to so I made up this story and didn't expect it to go as far as it did. . . . I don't know why I couldn't have done something different."[6]

Marie was prosecuted and publicly persecuted for her actions. She struggled with mental health problems in the years that followed and, at one point, contemplated suicide. Then, in 2011, detectives found pictures of her assault among the possessions of a man who ultimately pled guilty to twenty-eight counts of rape and other felonies. Marie's initial statement—that she'd been assaulted by a stranger while alone in her home—was true.

The criminal investigations division where Marie reported her case did not include a separate sex crimes unit. If it had, the detectives might have been familiar with the existing rape investigation protocols and what to expect. They would have known, for instance, that victims commonly present as calm after a sexual assault, often confuse details, and may recant their stories. Even if the investigators couldn't put themselves in her shoes, they would have at least realized that Marie's reaction was similar to that of other rape victims.

I can't help but imagine how different this woman's life might have been if, instead of being met with invalidation, the detectives had said things like, "It's normal to recall new details weeks down the line. Give us a call if anything comes up," or "Don't worry if you remember things out of order. That's common after a trauma," or "If you're thinking of recanting your story so we'll stop asking you to recall the assault you're desperately trying to forget, we get it and will leave you alone now."

When a person is having a normal reaction to abnormal circumstances, Equalizing can help them make sense of the reality they've found themselves in. The flip side is that in the absence of being "seen," they can easily start to lose sight of themselves.

When the Abnormal Situation Is Perfectionism

Perfectionistic standards are like rigged carnival games. They're presented as easy and within reach when they're actually impossible and unattainable. People who are expected by others, or expect themselves, to achieve perfectionistic standards are trapped in a nonsensical world where normal and difficult are confused with perfect and easy. Unable to achieve perfection, they're bombarded with messages that they're not thinking, feeling, or performing normally:

Everyone else manages to keep their house in order while working full-time and raising kids.

No one else has to work this hard just to get by.

None of the other moms have a hard time getting up with their kids in the morning.

Of course, we're all shackled by perfectionism to some extent. Those last three statements were pulled from my own perfectionistic self-talk. In a world of carefully crafted profiles and photoshopped everything, developing an accurate sense of "normal" is an uphill battle. The constant distortion makes Equalizing all the more critical. It not only validates people's reactions but also recalibrates their expectations.

My client, a physician I'll call Lou, once came to session with a familiar problem: he couldn't keep up with emails at his new job, and he was struggling to complete his patients' notes on time, partly because of the email overload. No problem, I thought. We discussed ways to streamline his documentation process and came up with a plan for him to speak with the director if all else failed. Well, all else failed, including his conversation with the director, who my judgmental mind desperately wanted to be cast as Cruella de Vil.

No, she told him, Lou could not get staff assistance in responding to patient emails; yes, all patient emails needed to be addressed by end of day; no, he could not get weekly admin time to attend to these tasks as is customary in most hospitals and could make up missed work on his own time. The director didn't validate any of Lou's concerns and instead seemed to suggest that he should get with the program. Still, the demands seemed unreasonable. How were any of the other doctors staying afloat? Lou didn't know. The director wasn't beloved by any means, but no one else was complaining about the expectations or workflow.

"Maybe it's the OCD," he said after months of not being able to make it home in time to put his kids to bed. Lou had a history of obsessive-compulsive disorder, which manifested in excessive checking. When we started working together, he would check to see if the oven was off, then recheck to ensure it was off, then rerecheck just to be positive, then . . . you get the point. At work, he used to compulsively go over orders and prescriptions he'd submitted, driven by the anxiety that he'd made a mistake. But that was all in the past. Lou responded positively to treatment and had been symptom-free for years.

"Are you checking again?" I asked. He didn't think so but was starting to doubt himself. I reminded him of the unrelenting anxiety and obsessive thoughts that drove his compulsions. He admitted that the mafia goons* were noticeably absent. But if it wasn't the OCD, what was it? Lou's situation was growing increasingly Kafkaesque. He began looking for other jobs.

Then one day his director was gone. Fired or quit, Lou wasn't sure which. There was a new director, and the first thing she did was to ask the doctors for anonymous feedback about their needs and pain points. Then she scheduled a meeting with them, which focused primarily on acknowledging the concerns everyone had raised about managing emails. It turns out Lou wasn't an outlier after all. He was part of a silent majority. His burnout and hopelessness weren't abnormal reactions to reasonable demands; they

---

* I sometimes refer to mental health symptoms as "mafia goons" because *that's what they are*—silent, menacing forces that lurk around the periphery of your life, cracking their knuckles and making neck-slitting gestures any time you start to enjoy yourself.

were normal responses to unrealistic expectations. Even though the new director didn't have any immediate solutions to the email problem, Lou abandoned his job search. He no longer felt overwhelmed with hopelessness and self-doubt; his oxygen mask was firmly in place. If you can do it, Equalizing is THE validation skill to use with someone who is being pummeled by perfectionistic standards. The question is whether or not you can pull it off.

EQUALIZING MISTAKES

Fortunately, there are only a few mistakes you can make when Emoting. The two biggies are (1) diminishing someone's experience, and (2) invalidating strongly held beliefs.

Mistake #1: Diminishing Someone's Experience

Equalizing to validate teens provides an excellent example of how this skill can backfire. Adolescence is chock-full of firsts—first loves, first jobs, pubic hair! These new experiences grab the table that the "normal" kids have been sitting at all their lives and flip it upside down. Because so much of what they're thinking, feeling, and doing doesn't *feel* normal, they don't necessarily want to hear that it is. Rather than validating the intensity and singularity of what they're going through, Equalizing can reduce it to common. This holds true for anyone who is responding to a new or intense situation.

If you're worried about diminishing someone's experience, all you need to do is validate the uniqueness of their situation. No matter how common it is, no two situations are exactly the same. Equalizing *and* validating the uniqueness of their situation allows you to demonstrate understanding without coming off like a know-it-all; adding the Caroline Qualifier also can help:

I've heard many divorced people say that being alone in the house at night takes some getting used to (Equalizing). *I imagine it's that much harder living out in the woods like you do* (validating the uniqueness of their situation). *I'm impressed you haven't booby-trapped your* *house,* Home Alone *style, and surrounded yourself with Dobermans* (Caroline Qualifier).*

Mistake #2: Invalidating Strongly Held Beliefs

You'll want to be mindful of invalidating strongly held beliefs anytime you're in the Kafkaesque land of perfectionism. People who are invalidating themselves for failing to meet perfectionistic standards often internalize those standards as normal. Telling someone who is convinced they're fat that their BMI is normal might *in*validate their tightly held perception of themselves. If a negative self-image is central to how an individual sees themselves, they're unlikely to feel seen by someone who challenges it.

You'll know if you've invalidated a strongly held belief because, well, the other person will act like you've invalidated them. Signs include them doubling down on their point, insisting, "You don't get it," and, if you're in an old-timey movie, slapping you in the face. If you run into these types of reactions, back up and try to Contextualize. Someone with a distorted perception of normal is responding from a place of conditioning, misinformation, or, in some cases, disorder. Remember, if a reaction doesn't make sense in terms of the current situation, try to find the context in which it does.

RECAP

- Equalizing communicates that a person's response is reasonable or justified in terms of the current situation and normal biological functioning. It's the "anyone in your shoes would do the same" skill.

---

*   In general, folks tend to play it too cautiously when it comes to validating emotions like fear or sadness because they're afraid of amplifying the other person's negative emotions. In reality, though, validation tends to bring down sympathetic arousal, unless the individual is already flooded (i.e., with a heart rate over 90 beats per minute) or highly distressed. If my friend were to call me when she's lying in bed at night alone and having a panic attack, then the Caroline Qualifier might hurt more than it helps. But if the individual isn't in an overwhelming state of distress, you shouldn't worry about acknowledging their emotions or the uniqueness of their situation.

- Like the other **Understanding Skills,** Equalizing comes down to logical reasoning and communication.
  - » Logical reasoning approaches:
    - › Default: Person's reaction = how people typically respond
    - › Golden Rule: Person's reaction = how I'd respond
  - » Communication:
    - › First-person: Saying that someone's reaction is equal to how *you* would react (use if you're an authority or peer).
    - › Third-person: Stating that their response is equal to how you imagine *others* would react (use if you don't know the person or situation well).
    - › Caroline Qualifier: Sweetens the standard Equalizing message of "anyone in your shoes would react similarly" with "and you're handling it better than most."
- Equalizing is critical when . . .
  - » Someone is having a normal reaction to an abnormal situation.
  - » The abnormal situation is perfectionism.
- Common mistakes associated with Equalizing include the following:
  - » Diminishing the other person's experience.
    Solution: Validate the uniqueness of their situation, or use the Caroline Qualifier.
  - » Invalidating strongly held beliefs.
    Solution: Take a step back and Contextualize or use the **Mindfulness Skills.**

PRACTICE TIP

Work on using the Golden Rule approach of putting yourself in someone else's shoes. When it comes to communicating your understanding, experiment with the first- and third-person approaches. Ideally, you'll be able to practice Equalizing daily this week, but if you can't, at least try putting yourself in another person's shoes. Note: don't assume you're strong in this skill just because you're emotionally intuitive or good at perspective taking. Understanding and communicating understanding are two different things.

Hint: Equalizing in combination with the Caroline Qualifier is a great way to reinforce young kids. Communicating that they're behaving more maturely, independently, etc., than you would have at their age is tantamount to giving them candy. For example: "I can't believe you got your chores done without me having to remind you. I would never have been able to do that at your age."

CHAPTER 10

PROPOSE—HOW TO READ MINDS

The most important thing in communication is hearing what isn't said.

—PETER DRUCKER, *A WORLD OF IDEAS*

Reader, I am your soulmate. I mean, I'm not, but if we spent enough time together, you might start to think I am. I'm not talking mystically or spiritually; by *soulmate*, I mean someone who seems to know you better than you know yourself and to whom you feel deeply connected. The validation skill Proposing can have just this effect. It communicates an understanding of someone's experience beyond what they've shared. I'm not actually the Yoko Ono to anyone's John Lennon; I'm just good at Proposing.

Technically speaking, Proposing means stating what you think another person is thinking, feeling, or wanting to do based on what they've said and what you know about the situation.* Proposing is often described as "mind reading," but it's more about reading between the lines. In the first chapter, when I described transitioning from problem-solving to validation with my suicidal client, I did so by Proposing:

---

* Other names for this skill include Read Minds, Articulate the Unverbalized, and Mind Reading. (Linehan, *DBT Skills Training*, "Handout 18"; Linehan, "Validation and Psychotherapy," 364.)

"This sucks," I said (Proposing a thought he might be thinking).

"You let your guard down for one second and are immediately attacked with questions from the overzealous graduate student you want to believe gives a shit but is most likely just doing what she's told" (Proposing a thought).

"And if that wasn't enough, the whole thing is being broadcast to a room full of people you've never met" (Proposing a thought).

Proposing can take some getting used to. I've personally worked on this skill more than any other on the Validation Ladder, and for good reason. That soulmate effect is something else. I talked a big game earlier about how if I used this skill on you it might make you feel deeply connected to me, but as is always the case with validation, these effects are not one-sided. I'd feel the connection as well. And although I know it's not exclusive to only one person in the universe as per the traditional soulmate trope, the connections this skill creates are no less meaningful.

HOW TO READ MINDS

By now, you know the drill: **Understanding Skills** can be broken down into logical reasoning and communication. With Proposing, you first have to draw some hypotheses about the other person's experience; then, you need to share your oh-so-educated guesses without insulting or, God forbid, invalidating them.

This skill isn't always difficult to pull off. Proposing "You must be exhausted" to someone who says they haven't slept in three days doesn't require a ton of interpersonal know-how. But you're not going to achieve that soulmate effect by pointing out the obvious. To harness the power of this skill, you need to be able to read between the lines and communicate your insights with just the right amount of confidence. Essentially, you've got to read people's minds without making them uncomfortable. I know, not exactly easy peasy lemon squeezy. This level of Proposing does require a fair bit of emotional intelligence (EQ), but here's the thing: unlike intelligence (IQ), which is hard to budge, EQ can be improved.[1] This is one of the many reasons I maintain that emotional sensitivity is an advantage when it comes to mastering validation skills, but not a requirement. The EQ needed for skills like Proposing can be developed by breaking down and practicing them. So let's get to it!

Logical Reasoning

If you want to figure out what another person is thinking, you need some information to go on. And what's the easiest way to get information on people? Go through their phones. I'm kidding. No, the best way to get info on folks for the purposes of Proposing is to use the **Mindfulness Skills.** Specifically, Attending by playing the A Game and asking questions. I'll let Elna Baker show you how it's done.

Baker is a producer for *This American Life,* a weekly podcast and public radio show. She's also got game when it comes to validation. In an episode titled "Rom-Com,"[2] Baker spoke with her friend, comedian Michelle Buteau, about an uncommon obstacle Buteau faced in her first serious relationship: after dating for three years and building a life with the man she hoped to marry (they later broke up), Buteau found out that he was illiterate. Having told versions of this story many times in her stand-up, Buteau is polished and entertaining, but Baker knows what she's doing. I've included a snippet of the interview below. See if you can spot the two validation skills Baker uses to add unexpected depth to the story and connect with Buteau.

> **Baker:** [explaining to listeners how Michelle began to resent her partner for refusing to get help]: Even when they were happy, she'd snap herself out of it and think, wait, no, no. We're forgetting that there's this huge, looming

problem, and we've got to fix it before everything can be OK. She started to resent him.

Buteau: We don't even laugh anymore. We're not even holding hands like we used to. We're not even having sex like we used to, simply because you're not going to this class. Like, if you just went to a class, I would just be so happy.

Baker: Did you feel like, if you love me, you will learn to read?

Buteau: Absolutely. I mean, is that weird? But I totally felt like that. I was like, who's going to read books to our kids at night? Like, you've got to get it together. This was like the bane of my existence. I was like—and I couldn't really talk to anyone about it, because how embarrassing. Because I didn't want my friends to think less of him, you know? And I wanted him to still feel like a man, so I just kind of carried this by myself. And at some point, I just looked at myself and I was like, you've got to go. But even then, it was just like, how do I leave somebody when they're down?

Baker: Well, in a sense, it actually, like, it made the relationship last longer because everything became about him reading. And so if you could just crack that or fix that, then maybe it would work out.

Buteau: Oh, my god, what are you? Dr. Phil with tits? [laughter]. Yeah, I mean, I feel like I always live like that. If I could just lose those twenty pounds . . . And so, yeah, there was that. You know, if we could just get past this, then we'll live the life we're supposed to live.*

Baker's interjections are brief but intentional: she uses Attending (**Mindfulness Skill**) to foster insights, which she then Proposes (**Understanding Skill**). Remember:

---

* Mat said this snippet makes Buteau sound like a jerk. She's not. At other points in the interview, she describes being heartbroken after learning about the circumstances that contributed to her ex-boyfriend's illiteracy and how she felt deeply committed to supporting him when they were together. Their inability to dialogue or work on the issue eventually drove them apart. Also, he cheated on her, so there's that.

Mindfulness → Understanding → Empathy

In the interview, after Buteau describes her growing resentment toward her boyfriend's complacency, Baker asks, "Did you feel like, if you love me, you will learn to read?" Baker's Attending question is bound to elicit more information about why this issue matters to Buteau, which will advance Baker's game. Girl clearly knows how to play! As predicted, Buteau gives Baker lots to work with, which Baker then uses to draw some connections. Rather than keeping her insights to herself, Baker risks Proposing them, "Well, in a sense, it actually, like, it made the relationship last longer. . . ." Buteau then exclaims, "Oh, my god, what are you? Dr. Phil . . . ?" If you listen to the audio recording, it's clear that Buteau isn't mocking her interviewer; she's impressed by her understanding. Baker highlighted something Buteau hadn't articulated. Baker is not just paying attention; she gets it. She gets it in a way Buteau maybe didn't until that moment. And there it is, that soulmate effect.

Springboarding off of the A Game is the most logical way to approach Proposing: you collect data, draw some hypotheses, and then run them up the flagpole to see if the other person salutes. But you also can use the Golden Rule approach of putting yourself in the other person's shoes to help you figure out what to Propose.

When I was struggling to connect with the suicidal client I described in chapter 1, I didn't rely on the A Game to turn on the light bulbs I needed to see what I should Propose; instead, I tried to look at the situation from his perspective. Seeing the word V-A-L-I-D-A-T-I-O-N on the monitor screen immediately cued me to stop focusing on my experience—my fear, my failure, my panic—so that I could consider his. As the therapist, I was thinking, "I'm losing him. What do I do?" If I were the client, being hammered with questions by a graduate student who has clearly been made anxious by my vulnerable disclosure, I'd think, "This sucks." I'd think, "You let your guard down for one second and are immediately attacked with questions from the overzealous graduate student you want to believe gives a shit but is most likely just doing what she's told."

As the therapist, being observed by her colleagues and supervisor, I was thinking, "They know I'm an idiot. They're gonna bust through the doors any minute to save this guy from me. I'm going to therapist jail, where I deserve to rot for my incompetence." As a client who feels exposed and wishes they could take back what they said, I'd think, "And if that wasn't enough, the whole thing is being broadcast to a room full of people I've never met." If I were my client, I'd want to leave. So that's what we did.

Communication

Imagine a dial with the word *Idea* on it. If you turn the dial to the left, your idea will be Proposed as a suggestion: for example, "Maybe you're tired of having to work so hard to please your mother-in-law?" Turn it the other way, and it's stated as a fact: for example, "You're tired of having to work so hard to please your mother-in-law." If you're going for effect or want to project confidence in your understanding, state your idea more as a fact. To convey deference or respect for the other person's experience, lean toward couching it as a suggestion. Note that roles, relationship dynamics, and cultural norms may also determine whether it's more effective to state ideas as suggestions or facts.

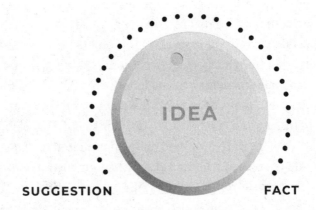

SUGGESTION   FACT

Lead-ins like "maybe," "I wonder if," and "it seems to me" are on the suggestion side of the Idea dial; they sound less intrusive, authoritative, and presumptuous. Framing insights as questions can also help you stay in suggestion territory. Saying, "Do you think you'd go back to working full-time if you didn't feel so guilty about leaving the kids?" sounds more curious and open to correction than, "You'd go back to full-time work if you didn't feel so guilty about leaving the kids."

Generally speaking, Proposing suggestions is the way to go if you're just getting to know the other person or if they're someone you need to show a healthy level of respect toward, like a mentor, manager, or Meghan Markle. I'm serious about Meghan Markle. When Oprah, the queen of Proposing, interviewed the former Duchess of Sussex, she knew to stick with suggestions. "Were you silent, or were you silenced?"[3] Oprah asked after Markle delicately tried to explain why she stayed mum when the media was spreading misinformation about her. This moment is the closest Oprah came to stating her insights matter-of-factly during their interview, but even at her boldest, she ticked her Idea dial ever so slightly toward suggesting by couching her point as a question.*

Proposing suggestions instead of facts works well when validating someone who is easily influenced, tends to doubt themselves, or presumes you know more than they do (e.g., children), because these sweet, trusting souls may be more likely to believe your perspective over their own.

Moving your Idea dial in the other direction by stating something as a fact is generally more powerful. With my suicidal client,

---

* Being the footnote-reading peruser you are, you might have noticed that "Attending Questions" and "suggestions Proposed as questions" seem like the same thing. They're not. Attending Questions are used to gather information and show that you're paying attention; suggestions Proposed as questions are intended to make a point to demonstrate understanding. Because we've got all the time and space in the world down here in the footnote, I want to take the opportunity to flag that Baker's question, "Did you feel like, if you love me, you will learn to read?" might actually have been intended to demonstrate understanding, rather than to gather more information. Given where she goes with it, I think it was a genuine question, but with a skilled validator like Baker, it can be hard to tell.

I said, "This sucks," not, "Maybe you're starting to feel like this therapy session sucks." In speaking to my friend's mom about her unraveling marriage, I said, "This is awful," not, "Does this feel awful?"*

Stating your points matter-of-factly gives weight to them. It says, "This is how things are," as opposed to, "Is this how things seem?" If what you Propose resonates with the other person, your certainty can take a sledgehammer to their doubt and insecurity. I'm reminded of a thirty-something woman in my group of mom friends who started crying and nodding emphatically when I said, "You must be devastated," after she told me her parents were divorcing. This woman was very close to her parents and had modeled her marriage after theirs. It seemed obvious to me that she'd be heartbroken by the news, but she apparently wasn't sure if it was reasonable for a married adult woman who no longer lived with her parents to be as upset as she was about them separating. By Proposing an emotion she hadn't surfaced, I communicated that her reaction was rational, understandable, and, as such, valid.

Proposing your ideas as facts implies some degree of certainty on your part. That degree can be amplified or reduced through Attending nonverbals (aka the Big Four: proximity, eye contact, gesturing, and nodding). The other evening, I had a clusterfuck of health stuff going on. I was in a lot of pain from a root canal earlier in the week, I had a yeast infection from the antibiotics I'd taken post–root canal, and I was scheduled for a three-hour medication infusion the next day, which would be followed by forty-eight hours of labored breathing and inhalers because I'm allergic to the treatment. To make a long story short (too late), I was a hot mess. My way of complaining to Mat about all this was to jokingly ask if he thought I could sway the nurse to put me in a medically induced coma for the next seventy-two hours, and if so, could he empty the dishwasher while I'm out? He didn't respond to my questions.

---

* In case you missed this, I shared this example in the introduction. But if you're reading the footnote, you probably read the introduction. You are my people.

Instead, he put down the iPad he'd been scrolling on and sat next to me on the floor. He placed his hand on mine, looked me in the eye, and said, "This is scary." Boom. I was shook. Mat is definitely the John to my Yoko. I was feeling scared. I don't know why: root canals and yeast infections aren't going to kill you, and I've been dealing with the monthly suffocation infusions for years, but still, I was scared. Mat could have said "This is scary" from the couch where he was sitting behind me while continuing to look at his iPad, but it wouldn't have registered with me in the same way. The validation impact of what he Proposed was communicated through his nonverbals (proximity, eye contact, and touch).

IDENTIFYING AND RECOVERING FROM MISTAKES

Babe Ruth had an impressive batting average of .342, meaning that when he was at bat, he hit the ball 34 percent of the time. Put another way, he struck out 66 percent of the time. His home run average was 8.5 percent.[4] He was one of the best in Major League Baseball history, but still, more than 90 percent of the time, he wasn't hitting homers. I'm not a huge baseball fan, but when I think of Babe Ruth, I think of grainy black-and-white videos of a man waving to fans as he walks the bases after hitting a ball out of the park, not someone who struck out more than he hit. When it comes to Proposing, the greats are a bit like Babe Ruth: their dazzling "home runs" overshadow the frequency of their strikes.

The tricky thing about Proposing is that, unlike in baseball, you won't necessarily know if you struck out. People might not think it's worth the emotional energy it would take to correct you when you're wrong. Or they might not want to risk hurting your feelings. Because it can take a couple of attempts before you Propose something that resonates with the other person, mastering this skill comes down to detecting and recovering from mistakes.

Recovering

You may not have to do any detective work to determine if the idea you Proposed was a swing and a miss; sometimes, the other person will just tell you. For instance, when I was talking with the nanny in the park and Proposed, "You must feel like you're always taking care of people," after she described her work situation, she was quick to exclaim, "No, I don't!"

If someone responds to what you Proposed by getting defensive, correcting you, or arguing, then you got it wrong or you surfaced something they're not ready to accept. In either case, the two of you are not on the same page. You need to better understand how they see things, but you can get there only if you stay in the conversation.

The easiest way to stay engaged after striking out is to go back to playing the A Game and using Attending questions and comments. For example, the other day, I Proposed, "Your body is utterly exhausted," to validate a client who was crying about having slept through an important nine a.m. meeting following several nights of insomnia. "No," she said thoughtfully, "I think I subconsciously wanted to avoid it." Reader, between you and me, I'm pretty sure her body collapsed in on itself after going a remarkable fifty+ hours without sleep, but that wasn't her take on the situation. Rather than force my point, I followed up with an Attending question: "That's interesting; why do you think you wanted to avoid the meeting?"

Perhaps she thought what I initially Proposed was a veiled criticism, like I was implying that she needs to focus more on sleep hygiene. Or maybe she didn't accept how much insomnia was affecting her. Or perhaps she was right and her subconscious was like one of those monsters from the Upside Down that forces the *Stranger Things* kids to turn on themselves. Regardless, my understanding was incomplete, so I needed to retreat to the **Mindfulness Skills.**

I have to warn you that returning to the A Game after striking out with Proposing can feel counterintuitive. If someone comes off as defensive, annoyed, or invalidated by what you Proposed, your feelings might get hurt, which will incline you to either push your point or disengage. Fight or flight. Overriding your instincts can take some getting used to, but knowing which emotions to look out for—namely, hurt, embarrassment, self-doubt, and various shades of frustration—will make you infinitely better at spotting and challenging the urge to cut and run.

Once you've gathered more information through the A Game, take another swing at Proposing or one of the other **Understanding Skills** or **Empathy Skills**. I've said it before, and I'll say it again: Oprah is the queen of Proposing, but even she makes a lot of mistakes. She recovers by quickly reverting to the **Mindfulness Skills**, but she doesn't let missteps deter her from trying again. Because you're familiar now with many of the validation skills she uses, I've copied the description I gave of her approach in chapter 5 and added the skill sets and specific skills she uses to Oprahfy people:

Oprah says something like, "That must have been frustrating" (**Understanding Skill**: Proposing). *The guest responds with a correction: "It wasn't frustrating. It was terrifying." Oprah takes a step back without missing a beat despite having whiffed her validation attempt in front of a live studio audience: "Terrifying. What was terrifying about it?"* (**Mindfulness Skills:** Copying + Attending). *She listens thoughtfully and maybe follows up once or twice to clarify something they said* (Attending) *or repeat it to them* (Copying). *Then, she steps it up again, offering some insight they hadn't articulated and checking to see if it resonates* (Proposing). *She might need to do this several times, but eventually, she nails it.*

Like Babe Ruth, Oprah's misses are quickly forgotten after she hits the validation equivalent of a home run.

Detect

Imagine you're talking to a friend who recently retired from her job as a high school English teacher. You ask how she's enjoying retirement, and she vaguely suggests that it's not going well. "I have lots of free time," she says. "More than I know what to do with. . . ." You start playing the A Game, and based on the information you gather, you suspect she's feeling conflicted about how much she misses her job when she "should" be enjoying her retirement. And there it is, a big fat Proposing opportunity. You decide to take it: "It's hard to process a loss everyone says you should be celebrating."

You were so much more confident that this Proposed idea would resonate before you said it. Now, you're not so sure. Your friend isn't giving any indication that she feels validated by what you Proposed. That said, she's also not getting defensive or correcting you. Her exact response was, "Hmm." Hmm?! What are you supposed to do with a hmm? Nothing, that's what. To figure out where you stand and how to proceed, you'll need to go back to reading between the lines, which, in this case, means reading her nonverbal behavior.

Those with a high EQ can do this naturally by tapping into the emotional spidey sense that allows them to identify and understand people's emotions. For everyone else, remember that EQ can be developed. You just need to know which emotional tells to look for and how to interpret them. Nonverbal signs that someone feels *validated* by what you Proposed include them doing the following:

- Maintaining or making eye contact.
- Becoming more excited—speaking faster or louder, using more physical gestures, appearing more animated.
- Leaning in or moving closer to you.

The less obvious but far more reliable indication of how someone feels about what you Proposed is their facial expression. I've heard it said that "the eyes are windows to the soul," but it should be, "facial expressions are windows to the soul." Less catchy, I know, but far more accurate. Even more precise would be to say that "micro expressions are windows to the soul, but you may only be able to see them for like a millisecond because people are quick to cover them up." Yeah, that's never gonna catch on.

Renowned facial expert Paul Ekman defines micro expressions as "facial expressions that occur within a fraction of a second."[5] According to Ekman, "This involuntary emotional leakage exposes a person's true emotions."[6] I had to quote him verbatim because there's simply no better way to say "emotional leakage" than "emotional leakage."

If you pick up on leaked negative emotions like disgust, fear, or contempt, then it's unlikely the other person feels validated by you. Not great at detecting emotional leakage? No problem. Ekman has developed a tool to help people get better at identifying and interpreting emotional leakage. It also can improve your ability to tell if someone is lying. So, you know, two birds, one stone. You can find versions of Ekman's Micro Expressions Training Tool on his website or via a link to it on mine.*

If you're all, "Caroline, I refuse to look up Ekman. You promised I'd find everything I needed in this book," then fine. I'll leave you with one last reliable way to tell if you failed or nailed your validation attempt. The tell is whether the person sticks with the conversation. If you did read their mind or, better yet, made a connection they hadn't, they'll want to extend the conversation. Validation feels good, and when something feels good, we want more of it. However, if what you Proposed made them feel awkward, uncomfortable, or invalidated, they won't be motivated to keep talking. Even people pleasers will want to get the hell out of there. They might throw you a thoughtful, "I hadn't looked at it that way," so you can feel satisfied with yourself, but they'll change the topic or abandon the conversation at the first opportunity. Similarly, if the other person has tried repeatedly to correct your understanding without success, they'll eventually feel punished out of continuing the conversation and will drop it.

---

* Paul Ekman Group, https://www.paulekman.com/micro-expressions-training-tools/.

The problem with relying on the Conversation Tell is that by the time you detect it, you might not be able to recover. Forcing a conversation with someone who has made it clear that they want to end it can make them feel unsafe. You should still attempt an Attending question or two after detecting the Conversation Tell, but be prepared to drop your agenda if they don't engage. If you think you might have really done damage by invalidating the other person, say so, and apologize for the offense.

Given how difficult it can be to recover from the Conversation Tell, I encourage you to rely on other nonverbal cues to the extent that you can. And if you can't because you struggle with detecting and interpreting nonverbals, you really should check out Ekman's tool, which is totally worth it when you consider the amount of time you put into learning things like long division, which you probably never use, compared to learning how to detect "emotional leakage," which you'll use constantly and might one day help you know for sure if the clerk at IKEA is lying when he says they don't have any more Billy bookcases in back before even checking.

RECAP

- Proposing means saying what you suspect another person is feeling, thinking, or wanting to do based on what they've said and what you know about the situation.
- As with the other **Understanding Skills**, Proposing can be broken down into logical reasoning and communication.
  - » Logical reasoning:
    - › Play the A Game and use Attending questions to help you gather the information you need.
    - › Use the Golden Rule approach of putting yourself in the other person's shoes.

» Communication:
  › To convey deference or respect, Propose your idea as a suggestion by using qualifiers like "I wonder if . . ." or framing your ideas as questions.
  › To project confidence, state your idea more as a fact; combining the Big Four Attending nonverbals with matter-of-fact statements increases the firmness of your message.
- To become a pro at Proposing, you must be able to recover from and detect mistakes.
  » Recover: Drop down to the **Mindfulness Skills**— Attending and Copying. Try Proposing again or use another **Understanding Skill** or **Empathy Skill** when you can.
  » Detect: Rely on your emotional intuition, look for nonverbal behavior or emotional leakage, or use the Conversation Tell.

PRACTICE TIPS

1. Like Attending, Proposing requires more repetition than some of the other skills to master. Twenty-five reps is a great target for this skill and will help you internalize all the finer points in this chapter that you're currently convinced you'll forget. For this week (and beyond if you're going for twenty-five reps), practice using the A Game and the Golden Rule approach to draw hypotheses about what someone might be thinking or feeling. Be sure to experiment with framing your ideas as *suggestions* and *facts* across different scenarios to get a feel for the difference. If Proposing makes you nervous, practice using it in low-stakes conversations about topics like sports, food, TikTok videos, etc., before attempting more serious or emotional discussions.

2. Check out Ekman's website for resources to help improve your ability to identify emotional leakage. If you suspect you're already good at leakage detection, check out his quizzes to know for sure. Then you can brag to all your friends about how high your EQ is, which won't be annoying at all. Just kidding, that would be super annoying, but if you have a high EQ, you already know that.

CHAPTER 11

TAKE ACTION—WHEN WORDS AREN'T ENOUGH

All of us, at some time or other, need help. Whether we're giving or
receiving help, each one of us has something valuable to bring to this world.
That's one of the things that connects us as neighbors—in our own way, each
one of us is a giver and a receiver.

—FRED ROGERS, *THE WORLD ACCORDING TO MISTER ROGERS*

As I write this, Russia is at war with Ukraine. People have fled the country in droves, and every day the world is overwhelmed with images of the war crimes committed against those remaining. Ukrainians do not have the military strength to fight Russia on their own. Their president, Volodymyr Zelenskyy, has been meeting around the clock with his nation's allies, pleading for economic sanctions, weaponry, and a no-fly zone over Ukraine. In a rare interview with ABC News that aired on March 7, 2022, President Zelenskyy was asked what message he wanted to send to the American people.[1] Zelenskyy spoke in Ukrainian and used a translator throughout the interview, but when asked this final question, he looked directly into the camera and responded in English:

I just want you to feel and understand what it means for us.
Because always, American people, they speak about freedom,
and they know what it is. And now, when you are looking at
Ukrainians, I think you feel what that means for us. So we are
not far from you. We are not far from you. And that's why,

*Americans, if you see and if you understand how we feel, like
how we fight against all the enemies for our freedom, support
us, and not only with words, with concrete direct steps.*

Zelenskyy is asking for help because he cannot manage the situation on his own. Responding to his request by taking "concrete direct steps" is the only way to sufficiently validate Zelenskyy and the people of Ukraine. He hopes that if Americans *see* and *understand* that the freedom his country is fighting for is the same freedom they value, they will be compelled to respond with empathy by Taking Action.

Taking Action means directly intervening on another person's behalf.* Rather than offering solutions, or talking someone through how they might solve a particular problem, Taking Action has you step in to solve it for them. It's the "put your money where your mouth is" skill, and, in some scenarios, it's the only way to show that "you're there, you get it, and you care."

As an **Empathy Skill**, Taking Action has you go above and beyond acknowledging (**Mindfulness Skills**) and thinking logically about someone's experience (**Understanding Skills**). It requires you to *invest* yourself in the situation. The **Empathy Skills** achieve the aims of the other skills you've learned so far and go one step farther, transforming you from an observer into an active participant.

Wait, Isn't This Problem-Solving?

Taking Action sounds a lot like something I warned you never to do when validating—problem-solve. Our natural inclination toward

---

* Taking Action is similar to what Marsha Linehan refers to as Functional Validation, which is not included among the validation skills taught to clients but is discussed in her various articles and chapters written for therapists. It also appears as Responding with Action in the Dialectical Behavior Therapy for couples literature. (Linehan, "Validation and Psychotherapy," 380; Kelly Koerner and Marsha M. Linehan, "Validation Principles and Strategies," in *Cognitive Behavior Therapy*, eds. William O'Donohue, Jane E. Fisher, and Steven C. Hayes [Hoboken: John Wiley & Sons, 2003], 229–37; Fruzzetti and Iverson, "Mindfulness, Acceptance, Validation," 186.)

solving problems means we usually have to inhibit the urge to Take Action, not lean into it. Yet here I am telling you that Taking Action is sometimes the most effective way to validate people. What the hell?!

Problem-solving and intervening to solve someone's problems (Taking Action) aren't technically the same thing. Suggesting actions a person might take (e.g., "Maybe you should redo your résumé before sending out more applications") is different from intervening on their behalf (e.g., "I redid your résumé for you; now maybe you'll get more bites"). Problem-solving is a more *passive* attempt to change someone's experience, while Taking Action requires you to *actively* invest yourself in the situation.

While all that is true, Taking Action *is* focused on change. On the surface, this might seem incompatible with validation, which is all about communicating acceptance. But by now, you've seen how acceptance and change give rise to each other and can coexist. That's not to say Taking Action is the best way to demonstrate acceptance. *It often isn't.* Like problem-solving, Taking Action when it's not warranted reveals that you don't really understand the other person's situation or why they're coming to you. For instance, it might be validating to Propose "This is so unfair to you" after your friend tells you how her substance-abusing brother keeps hitting her up for money; Taking Action by staging an intervention for her brother probably wouldn't be.

The thing about Taking Action is that, when warranted, it can be more validating than all the other skills combined. This skill is essentially a power tool. Like a chain saw or a nail gun, it overcomes the limitations of more basic tools, and you can't do some jobs without it. As with any powerful tool, though, if you don't know how to operate it or fail to do so with caution, you may destroy what you set out to build. The question then is, how do you know if intervention is warranted? Being able to discern when to intervene and when to sit on your hands is where the skill lies in Taking Action.

WHEN ACTIONS SPEAK LOUDER THAN WORDS

The main thing to consider before Taking Action is whether the person actually *needs* or *wants* you to step in. Note that it may be validating to Take Action even if someone doesn't technically need you to intervene. I mean, I *could* throw myself a party to celebrate the completion of my book, but I'd feel validated by Mat if he chose to throw one for me. (*Hint, hint!*) What follows are my tips on how to intervene on behalf of someone who can and cannot Take Action themselves.

They Cannot Take Action Themselves

In his interview, President Zelenskyy asked the United States to take "concrete direct steps" because his country cannot defeat Russia on its own. President Joe Biden could respond to President Zelenskyy by Attending and Copying, "Ah, 'concrete steps.'" He could Equalize, "I think most world leaders would want international aid, too," or Propose, "You must be upset that Russia invaded your country." He could even use the other two **Empathy Skills**—Emoting and Disclosing—but let's face it, anything short of intervening will fail to validate the people of Ukraine. Without Taking Action, every other skill on the Validation Ladder would come off as condescending.

In some small, not nearly the same but sort of similar way, you can relate to Zelenskyy's position. We've all been in situations in which we required actions, not words, to feel validated. We don't feel validated by elected officials who fail to Take Action, despite claiming that they take our concerns seriously. In relationships, we don't feel validated by people who fail to change behaviors that hurt us. If anything, it would be *in*validating if an unfaithful partner said all the right things but continued to cheat on you. We're also not validated by people who fail to take our concerns seriously enough to respond with the help we need. If you broke your leg and asked your partner to do the dishes until you can walk again, they could construct an epic validation poem incorporating all of the other skills in this book to validate your request. But if they don't do the dishes, their validation poem will probably just piss you off.

Unfortunately, it's not as simple as "when someone asks for help, help them" if the other person cannot do what they're asking you to do. The problem with Taking Action is that it can quickly turn you into something no one wants to be: an enabler.

Havana is eight years old, and I still usually say sure when she asks me to brush the knots out of her hair before bed because, let's face it, she *can't* do it herself. To be clear, hair brushing isn't like emptying the dishwasher, which she can do but will try to complain her way out of doing, or vacuuming, which she can do but isn't great at. She literally cannot get her comb through the dreadlock-caliber knots she has in her hair by the end of the day. Validating Havana's pain and frustration with words as she tries to brush them out just doesn't feel, well, validating. I also should admit that I usually end up pulling her hair back for her during the day because when she tries, it ends up falling out and getting even more tangled. *Sigh*. It's a vicious cycle, but it's also a bit of an excuse. The truth? My name is Caroline Fleck, and I'm an enabler.

At least, I can be when it comes to Havana. For the most part, I'm actually pretty good at staying on the side of validating and not enabling when asked to Take Action, but I'm human, and my kid is cute, so inevitably, I screw up and intervene when I shouldn't. When I am effective with this skill, it's because I've done the due diligence of asking myself three questions. They might not all apply, but I will feel more confident about Taking Action if I can answer no to those that do.

To Act or Not to Act: These Are the Questions (to Ask Yourself)

1. Does this person have the *resources* required to take whatever action is needed?
2. Would I be doing something they need to *learn* to do

for themselves? If so, are they capable of developing the necessary skills?

3. Does the action conflict with my *values*?

Try to think of a time when someone asked you to Take Action (maybe not in so many words), and you considered doing so, at least in part, to validate them. You can choose something from the past or a current scenario, as in my hair-brushing example. Now try answering the To Act or Not to Act questions for the situation.

	Havana Asking Me to Brush Her Hair at Night	A Friend Asking for GoFundMe Donations to Help Them Rebuild Their Home After It Was Destroyed by a Wildfire	President Zelenskyy Appealing to Americans to Take "Concrete Direct Steps" to Protect the People of Ukraine
Do they have the required *resources*?	Yes, she has a brush and arms.	No, they lost everything.	No, they don't have the resources or power to defend themselves.
Would I be doing something they need to *learn* to do for themselves? If so, are they capable of developing the necessary skills?	Yes, and yes. Hair maintenance is a life skill she needs to develop, and at eight, she's capable of developing this skill.	No, this isn't a matter of skill.	No, this isn't a matter of skill.
Does the action conflict with my *values*?	No, I value good hygiene.	No, I value acts of service and supporting my friends.	Maybe! It depends on who you ask and what "concrete direct steps" entail (e.g., taking in refugees versus potentially triggering a war with Russia by instituting a no-fly zone).
Should I Take Action?	No, she can and should learn to do this herself.	Yes, it might be appropriate to Take Action.	Maybe! Depends on the individual's values and action being taken.

Remember, you should only consider Taking Action if you can answer no to all the questions. For examples, see the following table.

Isn't that handy?! Of course, others factors like cost, feasibility, and personal bandwidth also might be important for you to consider. The To Act or Not to Act questions simply help you determine if intervening is warranted. If not, you risk either enabling overdependence by protecting people from the consequences they need to develop necessary life skills or compromising your self-respect.

Should you decide *not* to Take Action, don't presume the other person will be scarred for life. **Remember, a cardinal rule of validation is that you should only validate the valid.** If you think the individual is capable of Taking Action themselves, you shouldn't validate the belief that they can't by intervening. Sometimes a person's doubts are valid; occasionally, they're not. Believing in someone who doesn't believe in themselves can validate their capabilities and help them realize their potential.*

The first time my family went skiing, we took a class together to learn the basics. When Havana took her first fall, I instinctively dug my poles in the snow to fight my way over to her. The instructor, a suspiciously laid-back woman in her twenties, put an arm out, stopping me in my tracks. "It's cool, dude," she said. "She'll figure it out." "Thanks, *dude*, but it's not cool," I almost blurted out. As I struggled to determine if my mama bear instincts justified me knocking out this woman with my poles and breaking both of my legs to get to my kid, something surprising happened. Havana got up. She figured it out on her own and brushed herself off, and the look of pride on her face once she steadied herself showed what this meant to her. The instructor didn't validate Havana's self-doubt by intervening; instead, she validated my girl's competence, strength, and resilience by believing in her.

Okay, so the To Act or Not to Act questions will help you determine if you should consider lending a hand when someone asks

---

* Note that you could validate the other person's feelings (e.g., fear, frustration, anxiety), or behavior of asking for help given their belief that they are incapable, but you do not need to validate their belief by Taking Action on their behalf.

you to do something they cannot do themselves. But what if they haven't asked you to intervene? Time for a story that is guaranteed to make a lot of doctors and therapists nervous:

Once upon a time, long before the days of teletherapy, I had a client who spent months building up the courage to pursue a highly effective but mildly tortuous treatment for obsessive-compulsive disorder (OCD).* Unfortunately, around the time she decided to begin, I moved my office out of the city where I'd been seeing her and to a suburb of Seattle. She didn't have a car and had to take a series of buses to reach me. The closest stop—which I passed on my way to and from work—was two miles from my office, which meant she was spending four hours commuting and four miles walking to see me so we could exorcize her OCD demons.** She'd arrive at my office totally bedraggled and wet from Seattle's rain, looking less like the fighter she hoped to channel for our sessions and more like a defeated, irritable cat someone had forced into a shower.

She was my last client of the day, and by the time I left the office, she would be well on her way to the bus stop. Between the darkness and the fog, she couldn't see me passing her in my car, but I could see me. And I hated what I saw: someone who was allowing their position to prevent them from being a decent person. Like so many

---

* Exposure Response Prevention (ERP) for OCD is the treatment I'm referencing here, and despite being slightly tortuous, I cannot recommend it enough! The tortuous part is that clients in ERP have to confront their worst fears while blocking the compulsive behavior they typically use to cope. For instance, if you're afraid of germs, we might have you touch a toilet for an hour without being able to wash your hands after. Learning to tolerate exposure to anxiety-provoking situations without engaging in compulsions is how those with OCD overcome the disease. (Edna B. Foa, Elna Yadin, and Tracey K. Lichner, *Exposure and Response [Ritual] Prevention for Obsessive Compulsive Disorder: Therapist Guide* [Oxford, UK: Oxford University Press, 2012].)

** No other providers with expertise in this treatment had openings, so she wanted to continue working with me. I'm stepping up on my teeny tiny soapbox down here in the footnotes to say that we need to reckon with the crisis that is our mental health-care system. In 2021, 65 percent of psychologists in the United States said they had no capacity to see new patients. More than half of people who need mental health care do not receive it. As John Oliver astutely noted after reviewing these statistics in a 2022 segment of *Last Week Tonight with John Oliver* titled "Mental Health Care," "When people do reach out for help, we're not in a position to give it to them." Okay, stepping down now. (*Last Week Tonight with John Oliver*, season 9, episode 18, "Mental Health Care," created and hosted by John Oliver, produced by Whit Conway, aired July 31, 2022 on HBO.)

doctors, I'd had it beaten into my head that I could be sued for anything at any moment. This is why I wasn't offering to drive her to the bus stop I passed on my way home. Because a young woman walking in the dark on the side of a busy road wasn't my problem, but if she got in my car, she could be. What if I got in an accident, or she claimed I said or did something unethical while we were driving?

After just two weeks, she was ready to quit. Her symptoms were debilitating, and she was desperate to complete the treatment, but the commute, she said, "is killing me." I validated her using the **Mindfulness** and **Understanding Skills**. Then, I took a step up the Validation Ladder: "What if I drive you to and from the bus stop?" She looked at me like I'd slapped her in the face. "You'd do that?" Clinically speaking, this was a no-brainer—she could not receive the treatment she needed otherwise. In terms of human decency, it was a no-brainer. And ethically, I didn't have any significant concerns.* So, yeah, I was willing to moonlight as an Uber driver so she could get her therapy on. She cried and told me I had no idea how much my offer meant to her.

During the next fourteen weeks, I adjusted my schedule so I could pick her up when she arrived at the bus stop and drive her back after our session. We agreed not to talk about anything personal or treatment-related in the car, and for the most part, we just listened to The National. But as soon as we walked into my office and shut the door, it was go time. Whatever fight she'd lost in the beginning came back twofold when it was clear to her that I was fighting right alongside her.

Intervening to help someone who needs assistance but hasn't asked for it can be a powerful way to Take Action. In addition to demonstrating mindfulness, understanding, and empathy, it shows astute attunement** to the obstacles that might interfere

---

* There are many situations in which driving a client would be problematic, therapy interfering, or dangerous. Based on my discussion with her and the consultation I received from colleagues, I decided that, in this particular situation, the risk of her not receiving treatment was greater than the risk of us driving together for a few minutes each day.

** This really doesn't justify a footnote; I just wanted to flag that I love how the term *astute attunement* sounds. Really hoping it catches on . . .

with them asking for the help they need. Taking Action in these situations sends a strong message that the individual's suffering is real and their need for support is valid.

The problem with Taking Action when someone hasn't asked you to intervene is that you might make the situation worse. This usually results from misreading social cues. The person can't take whatever action is needed, but they also don't want your help, thank you very much.

Several years after founding a start-up, my friend was tickled when her niece, Sam, decided to join the company as an intern. When my friend checked in with Sam following the first week of the internship, she expected to hear a glowing review of the company culture, which she'd been watering with diversity, equity, and inclusion initiatives and monthly off-sites. Instead, Sam told her that the company's lack of a unisex bathroom was disappointing. Sam, who is nonbinary, also said they found the bathroom signs—an alien in pants designating the men's room and one in a dress representing the women's—a bit tone-deaf. My friend felt terrible. She was the one who found the bathroom signs through a vendor on Etsy. And up until that moment, she thought they were the cutest things ever! Because the bathrooms were single-occupancy, she realized there was no reason for them to be gender-specific. That evening, she went home, purchased tasteful "All Gender" restroom signs, and installed them within a week. Then she received an email from Sam, saying they were upset and wanted to talk. You can probably see where this is going. Sam did *not* appreciate the signage swap. They were a newcomer in a pre-dominantly female company. The new signs went up soon after they started, which meant all signs pointed to them as the nonbinary person who'd taken issue with the cute aliens. Not a great first impression.

Condescending, patronizing, presumptuous—these are just some of the ways you can come across if you Take Action when someone doesn't want you to, despite lacking the skills or authority to intervene themselves. I'll say it again: the higher you go up the

Validation Ladder, the more it hurts when you fall. If you misread the interpersonal tea leaves and intervene where you're not wanted, you can end up invalidating the other person and feeling misunderstood by them in the process. Fortunately, there's a simple way to offset the chances of validation disaster in this situation: **Ask before you act.**

Had I pulled up creepily next to my client walking in the rain one evening, rolled down my window, and said, "Get in," in a throaty Batman voice, my attempt to Take Action might not have gone over so well. On the flip side, had my friend asked if her niece wanted her to change the bathroom signage, she could have demonstrated concern without crossing a line.

If you squirrel away a bunch of money so you can buy your wife a sports car to replace the oversized sedan she's always complaining about, you're acting before asking.* If you confront your kid's teacher about something that happened in the classroom after your kiddo confided in you, you're acting before asking. And if you spend the weekend completing a project your colleague can't finish because they're out with the flu, you're acting before asking. For the record, none of these examples were made up, and in each, the "benefactor" felt annoyed, not validated.

We're all too quick to put on our capes and come to the rescue of the people we care about, but in doing so, we often create more problems than we solve. The key to effectively Taking Action when the other person can't is to do it sparingly and mindfully. Ask yourself the To Act or Not to Act questions to see if Taking Action is appropriate and, if possible, ask the person if they want you to intervene first.

They Can Take Action Themselves

If friends and family hadn't brought us dinner a few times a week right after Havana was born, we would have been able to fend for

---

* If your name is Mat Fleck, please feel free to act without asking under these circumstances.

ourselves. We might have resorted to cereal if things got desperate, but there's no way I would forgo dinner after burning so many calories breastfeeding all day. Momma's gotta eat! And I would have. But when my mother-in-law, Rosa, snuck in to leave me my favorite casserole and then quickly ducked out so I didn't feel the burden of having to entertain while balancing a newborn on my boob, boy, did I feel seen (which I now realize is ironic, because she was intentionally trying not to see me). By honoring my unspoken desire for privacy and support, Rosa communicated that my needs were valid and that she at least was "there, got it, and cared." I felt similarly seen when my mom insisted on flying in a week before I was supposed to be induced. Her action assured me that the stress and fatigue I was feeling were real and that the situation warranted support, even if I could have survived without it.

Intervening when help isn't strictly necessary and hasn't been requested, as my loved ones did, reflects that astute attunement I mentioned earlier and can create a "How did they know?" reaction in the other person. *How did they know* I felt overwhelmed and would be relieved to have them pick up the kids? *How did they know* I was dreading pulling together those presentation slides? *How did they know* today was stressful and all I wanted was to come home to a pizza? (Side note: pizza is my comfort food. Mat knows this about me and has the uncanny ability to detect when I've had a hard day at work and want nothing more than to come home to a Chicago-style deep dish. Seeing that pizza immediately validates my emotions, need for comfort, and belief that Mat is the man of my dreams.)

Of course, because going above and beyond is more validating when it lands, it's all the more *in*validating when it doesn't. Ever encountered a situation in which someone who "just wanted to help" was making things worse? That's this skill gone sideways. Busybodying, overstepping, and boundary-pushing are the consequences of being too extra when it comes to doing things people can do for themselves.

The solution to the busybodying mistake is a two-parter. First, read the room. If you have any doubts about how others will receive your actions, **ask before you act**. Second, stay tethered to your intention. If your involvement creates conflict, it's not validating or caring; it's self-serving and harmful. Rather than getting defensive, doubling down, or playing the "They're so ungrateful" tape in your head, take a step back and remember why you were intervening in the first place. With validation, your intention is to show that you're there, you get it, and you care. If you're detecting signs of strain, you can remain mindful and understanding and show that you empathize by backing off without judgment.

Note: if people expect you to Take Action because *you always do*, you're not validating them; you're being taken for granted. You also might be depriving them of the opportunity to strengthen the skills they need to get better at managing their lives. You can get a sense of the effect this skill is having by observing how the other person reacts. Gratitude, "How did you know?" expressions, and heartfelt *thank-you*s suggest your action was validating. Lack of acknowledgment, entitlement, or demandingness means this skill might be working against you. Yes, you aim to validate someone, not get a ticker-tape parade for your efforts, but if the person treats you worse over time, or you don't feel good about yourself after intervening, back way off of this skill.

I want to close by noting that Taking Action isn't always about providing help. Investing your time by, say, reading that article your brother emailed you or listening to the podcast your friend keeps telling you to check out is among the easiest ways to validate through action. Sure, your partner can go to the school board meeting themselves, but if they ask you to go, validate their desire for support by joining them. Going a little bit out of your way will go a long way toward showing that you're emotionally attuned to the people around you.

RECAP

- Taking Action means directly intervening on another person's behalf.
- The main thing to consider before Taking Action is whether the other person actually needs or wants you to step in.
  - » When the other person *cannot* Take Action themselves:
    - › Ask yourself the To Act or Not to Act questions, and be sure you can answer no to each of them:
    - 1. Does this person have the *resources* required to take whatever action is needed?
    - 2. Would I be doing something they need to *learn* to do for themselves? If so, are they capable of developing the necessary skills?
    - 3. Does the action conflict with my *values*?
  - » If they haven't requested help, ask before you act.
- When the other person *can* Take Action themselves:
  - » Read the room, stay tethered to your intention, and be prepared to back off at the first sign of stress.
  - » If, over time, the other person acts entitled or becomes demanding, stop using this skill.

PRACTICE TIPS

Much of the intention and awareness required to Take Action effectively can be developed through reflection. Consider the following questions this week:

1. What are some ways in which you are currently Taking Action in your relationships? Note if the person can or cannot Take Action themselves.

2. What are some ways you have Taken Action in the past? Again, note if the person could or could not Take Action themselves.

3. How might you Take Action to validate the people you care about? You guessed it: note if the person can or cannot take whatever action you're considering.

4. How do others currently Take Action to validate you?

5. How have others Taken Action to validate you in the past?

For the scenarios above in which you identified Taking Action on behalf of someone who cannot or couldn't, ask yourself the To Act or Not to Act questions. If you are a parent, or tend to find yourself in codependent relationships, I'd recommend making an image of the To Act or Not to Act questions the wallpaper on your phone, or adding them to your list of potential forearm tattoos.

CHAPTER 12

EMOTE—MY ADVICE FOR JIMMY KIMMEL

I do not ask the wounded person how he feels,
I myself become the wounded person.

—WALT WHITMAN, "SONG OF MYSELF"

On June 11, 2019, at a House Judiciary subcommittee hearing on funding for the September 11th Victim Compensation Fund (VCF), Jon Stewart delivered an impassioned speech to a row of empty chairs representing the men and women of Congress who chose to skip the hearing.[1] His testimony, which quickly went viral, managed to expertly validate the first responders sitting and standing behind him while holding Congress accountable for their failure to do so. Take a look:

> *I want to thank Mr. Collins and Mr. Nadler for putting this together. But, as I sit here today, I can't help but think what an incredible metaphor this room is for the entire process that getting health care and benefits for 9/11 first responders has come to. Behind me [is] a filled room of 9/11 first responders. And in front of me, a nearly empty Congress. Sick and dying, they brought themselves down here to speak—to no one. It's shameful. It's an embarrassment to the country. And it is a stain on this institution. And you should be ashamed of yourselves for those that aren't here, but you won't be because*

accountability doesn't appear to be something that occurs in this chamber.

We don't want to be here. Lu [Detective Luis Alvare] doesn't want to be here. None of these people want to be here. But they are, and they're not here for themselves. They're here to continue fighting for what's right. Lu's going to go back for his 69th chemo. The great Ray Pfeiffer would come down here, his body riddled with cancer and pain, where he couldn't walk, and the disrespect shown to him and to the other lobbyists on this bill is utterly unacceptable.

You know, I used to get . . . I would be so angry at the latest injustice that's done to these men and women and, you know, another business card thrown our way as a way of shooing us away like children trick-or-treating, rather than the heroes that they are and will always be. Ray would say, "Calm down, Johnny. Calm down. I got all the cards I need." And he would tap his pocket . . . where he kept the prayer cards of 343 firefighters. The official FDNY [Fire Department of New York City] response time to 9/11 was five seconds. Five seconds! That's how long it took for FDNY, for NYPD [New York City Police Department], for Port Authority, for EMS to respond to an urgent need from the public. Five seconds. Hundreds died in an instant. Thousands more poured in to continue to fight for their brothers and sisters.

The breathing problems started almost immediately. And they were told they weren't sick—they were crazy. And then, as the illnesses got worse and things became more apparent, "Well, okay, you're sick but it's not from the pile." And then, when the science became irrefutable, "Okay, it's the pile—but this is a New York issue. I don't know if we have the money."

And I'm sorry if I sound angry and undiplomatic, but I'm angry—and you should be, too; and they're all angry as well. And they have every justification to be that way. There is not a person here, there is not an empty chair on that stage that didn't tweet out, "Never forget the heroes of 9/11"; never forget their bravery; never forget what they did, what they gave to this country." Well, here they are! And where are they? And it would be one thing if their callous indifference and rank hypocrisy were benign. But it's not. Your indifference cost these men and women their most valuable commodity: time. It's the one thing they're running out of.

Stewart's use of validation throughout his statement is masterful. It would be difficult for anyone, regardless of their views on the VCF, to deny that Stewart has born witness to the first responders' stories, understands the obstacles they're facing, and empathizes with their cause. He succinctly communicates all of this in just a few minutes, without ever deviating from his goal of advocating on their behalf. Because he isn't addressing the First Responders directly, you might need to reread the transcript to identify the validation skills Stewart uses. He manages to incorporate all eight of them, but the two most responsible for his validation going viral are Taking Action,* which we discussed last chapter, and Emoting, which we turn to now.

Emoting means openly expressing your feelings—specifically, the feelings you have in response to what someone has shared with you.** You don't need to exaggerate your emotions; on the contrary, Emoting is all about authenticity. It's dropping whatever facade you're maintaining and allowing yourself to have an unfiltered, genuine response to another person. In Stewart's case, this meant abandoning the comedic persona people have come to expect from him. For others, it might mean leaning into playfulness. If you've ever been accused of taking yourself too seriously, you should give this one a try. You'll inevitably discover that when you

---

* Stewart Took Action by using his star power and oratory skills to raise awareness for the VCF and hold Congress responsible for their inaction.

** There is not an equivalent for Emoting in Linehan's Levels of Validation. It's closest in nature to her Level 6: Show Equality, but there are meaningful differences between the two. (Linehan, *DBT Skills Training*, "Handout 18.")

allow yourself to be as you are without pretense or posture, you create opportunities for others to do the same.

I rely heavily on this skill in my work with clients. Between previous experiences with therapists and depictions of them in the media, folks often come to therapy with the assumption that I am or think I am superior to them. (My cat can confirm that I am, in fact, *not* superior to anyone.) Unfortunately, nothing shuts down vulnerability and collaboration faster than an air of superiority and judgment. For this reason, I'm often intentional about expressing my genuine reactions to the experiences people share with me. In other words, I'm intentionally unintentional. When a client said they'd decided to run for public office, I jumped out of my chair and clapped. (I really thought this was a good idea!) When another told me about an embarrassing sexual experience from the previous night, I covered my eyes with my hand and smiled. And when someone excitedly reported that they'd asserted themselves in a meeting and succeeded in changing the direction of a major project despite being a junior team member, I exclaimed, "You've got to be shitting me!" These reactions, although definitely not the most dignified, represent my natural inclinations in these moments. Rather than censoring my emotions, I shared them openly. In doing so, I went a step beyond engaging and thinking about the experiences shared with me; I allowed myself to be genuinely and transparently affected by them.

By this point, I hope I've convinced you that you don't need to be a psychologist to use skills like Emoting on the regular. Tearing up when someone shares a touching experience they had is an example of Emoting. Shuddering and making gagging sounds when your kid tells you about something gross also counts as Emoting. And if an IKEA employee was to say they're "frustrated by their company's ineptitude" after your shipment got delayed thirteen times, that would be yet another example of Emoting, but that of course would never happen. The point is, there's plenty of opportunity to use this skill, and IKEA should either require validation training for their employees or stop selling items they don't have in stock.

HOW TO GET REAL

Emotions can be complicated and scary, but Emoting doesn't have to be. It can be achieved through one of three modes of expression: nonverbal behavior, labeling, or implying.

Nonverbal Behavior

The Big Four nonverbals you learned for Attending—eye contact, proximity, gesturing, and nodding—demonstrate engagement. They show that you're paying attention, but they don't really reveal your feelings. Emoting nonverbals, on the other hand, do. They are wordless expressions of emotion that indicate not only that you're paying attention but also that you're affected by what the other person is saying. This might seem like a small distinction, but it has big consequences. Have you ever discussed or presented an issue you care about to a group? If so, then you know the distinction between people who are politely following along with what you're saying and those who are *feeling* it. Knowing that people are paying attention to you when you're talking is nice. Seeing that they understand and care is *awesome*.

Given that we have lots of emotions and ways of expressing them, I don't have a short list of nonverbals you should focus on. Nonverbals used to Emote can be as subtle as a hand to the heart in response to something touching, a jaw dropped in surprise, or a slow headshake to show disbelief. They can be dramatic, like jumping up and down in excitement, pounding a fist in frustration, or actually crying. If you watch Jon Stewart's speech, you'll see his lips quiver and eyes tear up when he says, "Your indifference cost these men and women their most valuable commodity: time. It's the one thing they're running out of." His words are powerful, yet it's his nonverbals that reveal the emotion behind them. And it is his emotion in this moment that communicates how much he empathizes with the first responders he's representing.

Rather than trying to do anything specific when Emoting, focus instead on letting down your guard and leaning into your emotions as they arise. Emoting is a natural extension of the Golden Rule approach I discussed in the **Understanding Skills**. Putting yourself in another person's shoes helps you connect with their emotions. Allowing yourself to uninhibitedly experience and embody those emotions is a way to demonstrate the empathy you're genuinely experiencing.

Although I do encourage you to make use of nonverbals, I don't mean to suggest that you should exaggerate them. Emoting stops being effective the moment it appears contrived. And there's really no reason to fake it, because we are all hardwired to show our emotions nonverbally as we experience them. Babies aren't trying to please us when they squint their eyes and smile—their sweet little baby nonverbals are an unconscious indication of their genuine delight.

What's confusing about nonverbal expressions is that although they are initially involuntary, our environments quickly teach us to control them. The little snow globes we occupy provide us with all sorts of direct feedback (e.g., "Carlos, when you lose the spelling bee, you should smile graciously and shake hands with the winner, not stomp your foot and cry") and indirect feedback (picture kids laughing and pointing at little Carlos as he cries) about the appropriateness of our nonverbals. This feedback makes us more aware and ultimately better able to control them. Eventually, we don't need to think about masking our emotions; we do it automatically.

But here's the thing—the feedback we've internalized about what is and isn't appropriate may not have been accurate, or might not apply to the situations we find ourselves in today. Invalidating messages like "Boys don't cry" and "Don't be so dramatic" not only are hurtful in the moment; they also discourage us from expressing the emotions associated with these criticisms in the future. We bottle ourselves up so quickly and tightly that even the thought of experimenting with Emoting can feel unnatural, if not outright dangerous. Unfortunately, in the absence of experimentation, we're unlikely to receive the feedback required to adapt our behavior over time to better suit our current environment.

Labeling

An obvious way to communicate your emotions is to label them. Labeling is as direct as you can get, but direct doesn't have to mean intrusive or distracting. Consider Stewart's statement: "I'm sorry if I sound angry and undiplomatic, but *I'm angry.*" He labels his emotion plainly but just as quickly draws attention away from himself and back to the main issue: "and you should be, too; and they're all angry as well. And they have every justification to be that way."

When stating how you feel, be sure to stick with *emotion* adjectives—sad, angry, disappointed, excited, relieved, etc.—rather than thoughts, as you do when implying emotions (see below). And remember, your aim is to support the other person, not draw attention away from them.

Implying

Last but not least, you can Emote by stating thoughts that imply emotions. You might say, "What a jerk!" to show that you're angry about how someone was mistreated, or "Spit it out already" to express anticipation, or even, "I just peed a little," which is what my best friend said in excitement when I told her I'd gotten engaged. Implying emotions allows you to incorporate humor (always a plus) and can be less jarring than stating your feelings outright, especially if the other person is "emotion-phobic."* Implying offers a safe, "we can talk about feelings without talking about feelings," approach to Emoting.

For instance, my dad can be overcome with emotions on your

---

* *Emotion-phobic* is a totally made-up term for the totally real fear some people have of identifying and expressing their emotions, often coupled with an inability to do so.

behalf, but he's not going to bust out an emotion wheel to help him articulate his feelings. He's a big "you've got to be kidding me" guy. "You've got to be kidding me" can mean he's excited by good news you've shared, frustrated by a setback you're telling him about, or surprised that you scored front-row seats to the Pistons. Don't get me wrong, dude has emotions, but he's a West Point grad turned Army veteran who was raised in the 1950s. Words like *disappointed* and *ecstatic* are not in his vocabulary.

So when my dad called to tell me that he needed to have a cancerous lump removed from his vocal chords—they caught it early and he has since fully recovered—I didn't use adjectives like *sad* or *scared* to validate him. I said, "You've got to be kidding me." This is the language he's most comfortable speaking. It's not that he wouldn't have understood what I meant if I had labeled my emotions; he just wouldn't have known what to do with them or how to respond. As Nelson Mandela is often quoted as saying, "If you talk to a man in a language he understands, that goes to his head. If you talk to him in his own language, that goes to his heart."* [2]

As for which mode of Emoting works best—nonverbal behavior, labeling, or implying emotion—it really depends on the situation. Nonverbals are great in circumstances in which talking would be inappropriate (e.g., weddings, funerals, graduations); you obviously can use them with implying and labeling emotions as well. Whether to imply or label will depend on how direct you want to be and the preferred "language" of the person you're validating.

WHEN TO GET REAL

As always, you should go as high up the Validation Ladder as you can without compromising authenticity, so some type of genuine emotional reaction is necessary to use this skill effectively. Beyond

---

* Mandela actually said, "Because when you speak a language, English, well, many people understand you, including Afrikaners, but when you speak Afrikaans, you know you go straight to their hearts."

that, Emoting can be a particularly powerful validation skill in situations in which you or the other person is "playing it cool" or inhibiting certain emotions.

They're Playing It Cool

People tend to play it cool when sharing vulnerable emotions like disappointment or when describing something that might be upsetting to another person. Even positive emotions like glee and excitement sometimes feel vulnerable because they can expose a person to judgment. In some ways, playing it cool by restraining emotions is an adaptive strategy—it allows people to evaluate if the person they're confiding in is safe and comfortable with the conversation topic. Although this strategy may protect folks from judgments and awkward conversations, it also can deeply misrepresent their true experiences. **By embodying the emotions another person is restraining, you can provide much-needed validation to someone who otherwise would not receive it.**

A few years back, a college friend I'd lost touch with reached out to say she'd moved to California. We were never best friends, but I liked her a lot and was sorry we hadn't stayed in touch. We met up for lunch, and as we got to talking, she mentioned that she hadn't worked in almost ten years since being "let go" by her previous employer. It didn't seem right to let it go at "let go." When I gently inquired about the circumstances surrounding her termination, she told me matter-of-factly that her manager had tried to force himself on her and threatened to fire her after she resisted. He followed through on his threat, and she was let go several weeks later after continuing to deny his advances. She told her story as though she were reading it from a newspaper, with little expression or intonation. Rather than Copying my friend's flat tone and affect, I allowed my face to naturally pucker while I shook my head— nonverbal behavior indicating disgust and dismay—and said something to the effect of, "I'm so disgusted. No wait, I'm pissed. Nope, I'm equal parts disgusted and pissed" (labeled emotion). "He should be in jail right now, but I'm guessing he's probably president of the company" (implying feelings of injustice, indignation, and incredulity, while transferring the focus from me back to her).

"CFO!" she said, nodding her head and widening her eyes. She went on to share the aftermath of what happened following the termination, how it affected her then and affected her still. After our lunch, she followed up with an email thanking me for "listening to her story." She said it felt good to share it. Had I just focused on being mindful by Attending or Copying, I doubt she'd have reached out to thank me. But by channeling my inner Jon Stewart, I was able to "see" her and communicate that, as far as I was concerned, she had nothing to hide.

You're Playing It Cool (for No Reason)

You playing it cool is the inverse of the situation described above. In this case, you're the one having an emotional reaction to another person's experience, and you're intentionally trying to suppress it like Jimmy Kimmel. Yeah, the late-night host. See, Kimmel is a self-proclaimed crier. He's admitted to pinching his hand to keep himself from tearing up during heartfelt moments on air. But he isn't always successful. The ironic thing is that although Kimmel tries hard to play it cool, some of the most popular episodes of *Jimmy Kimmel Live!* are the ones in which he validated the seriousness of an issue or the suffering of others by Emoting.

After his newborn son required emergency open-heart surgery, Kimmel went on the air to share his experience and was moved to tears while discussing the reality of families who cannot afford health insurance. "If your baby is going to die and it doesn't have to, it shouldn't matter how much money you make . . . I saw a lot of parents there [in the NICU], and no, no parent should ever have to decide if they can afford to save their child's life," Kimmel said while openly crying.[3] I don't think people are rewatching and sharing this segment to make fun of the former host of *The Man Show* for crying on national television; episodes like these are popular for the same reason Stewart's clip went viral—because Empathy is contagious. Seeing someone moved to emotion on behalf of another person not only validates that person but also inspires empathy in others.

I'm not going to pretend that there aren't plenty of good reasons to hold back your emotions when validating another person (see my next section, "Emoting Mistakes"), but most of us are operating off of assumptions that don't always apply. We've internalized rules like "don't make it about you" and often presume that expressing our emotions will overwhelm or upset people. Although these are generally safe rules to live by, they're also incompatible with the **Empathy Skills**. The ability to use and establish a connection through the highest levels of validation is tantamount to what great poets and writers do. Breaking the rules, experimenting with form, and defying expectations elevate the language of validation to an art in which deep, intellectual, interpersonal, and intrapersonal connections are possible.

EMOTING MISTAKES

You can Emote through nonverbal behavior, labeling, and implying your emotions. Emoting can convey a strong signal of empathy and is a particularly effective skill to use when you or the other person appears to be downplaying emotions for no good reason. Of course, the more validating skills are also the easiest ones to mess up. Again, there are myriad cultural and contextual norms around Emoting that may cause it to backfire, the details of which are beyond the scope of this book. But I do want to highlight three Emoting mistakes you should avoid regardless of the context: coming on too strong, striking the wrong chord, and losing control.

Coming On Too Strong

The goal of validation is to communicate that you understand and empathize with the other person's experience. If your reaction is significantly more intense than theirs, it *might* indicate that you're not really attuned to their experience. Having a dramatic emotional reaction also can overshadow or "steal the thunder" of the person you intend to validate. Worse yet, if the other person is in fight, flight, or freeze mode, expressing your intense emotions can quickly overwhelm the situation. There's a reason first responders speak in a low, steady tone and provide reassurance in crisis situations—they know that expressing any anxiety, doubt, or fear would do more harm than good.

Striking the Wrong Chord

Expressing emotions that conflict with what the other person is actually feeling can create an immediate disconnect. You might, for example, giggle at what you mistook for mild embarrassment but was, in fact, deep humiliation, or express frustration that is discordant with somebody's grief. Unfortunately, if the other person cannot relate to the emotions you're expressing, they're unlikely to trust that you can relate to theirs.

Losing Control

In truth, losing control of one's emotions when Emoting happens far less than people fear, but it is worth mentioning. I once met with a mother whose fifteen-year-old had attempted suicide while in "treatment" for depression at a therapeutic boarding school. Suffice it to say that the treatment was a total sham and involved some questionable, if not unethical, approaches. The child returned home after the attempt, and her mother was looking for a new provider. I am a staunch advocate of evidence-based care and an expert in treating self-harm and suicidal behavior. I not only felt angry on behalf of this family; I also felt sad—*really* sad. The system had failed, if not exploited, them, and another bright young girl nearly lost her life in the process. The mother was tearful throughout our session, and in my attempts to validate her grief, I allowed myself to tear up as well. Except I didn't just tear up, I started crying. Like, straight up crying. I completely surprised myself, and the mom, too, based on her wide-eyed expression. I spend most of most days talking about suicide, trauma, and suffering. I'd heard versions of this mother's story countless times, and the idea that I'd lose my composure if I leaned into my emotions never crossed my mind. But for whatever reason, that day the work got to me. I was able to compose myself quickly enough and apologize, but the mom's emotions were noticeably muted after that. Far from validating her, my attempt at Emoting clearly shut her down. I'd never made this mistake before and haven't since, despite my ongoing use of this skill. Unless you repeatedly lose control of your emotions, I encourage you not to give up on Emoting, even if you happen to make this mistake.

MANAGING MISTAKES

To review, the three mistakes you want to be mindful of when Emoting are coming on too strong, striking the wrong chord, and losing control. Now for how to prevent and recover from these errors.

Prevention

The safest way to avoid making the mistakes mentioned above is through experimentation. Try expressing a toned-down version of your emotions, and see how the other person reacts. If they appear to loosen up and talk more, you might experiment with more intensity, presuming you can do so authentically. And although you shouldn't presume that your feelings will overwhelm somebody who is upset or down, you should be careful about expressing them to someone who is highly distressed or in crisis. Finally, if you are deathly afraid of losing control, experiment first with Emoting positive feelings like excitement, enthusiasm, or pride, rather than negative feelings such as frustration or despair.

Recovery

If your emotions appear to make the person uncomfortable, shut down, or nervous, put aside your emotions and, as always, drop down to the **Mindfulness Skills**. Try asking an Attending question or two to reengage them and spend some time on your A Game before attempting another **Understanding Skill** or **Empathy Skill**. If the other person tries to change topics, let them; this shows that you're in control of your emotions and they're in control of the conversation. And as is always the case with laughing at yourself, if you can do it, do it! A simple, "I *clearly* need to cut back on my coffee" can go a long way.

If you happen to have the rare experience of losing control of your emotions, don't be hard on yourself. Remember, the point of validation is to communicate that you are there, you get it, and you care. It is our ability to be present for the other person that is compromised when our emotions overwhelm us. You can recover by circling back with them after you're composed. Try connecting by email or text messaging, if you don't trust your ability to stay collected in person, but—and hear me on this—you have to circle back. And don't just do it to check the "I circled back" box. Your friends and family will be all too quick to say it's no big deal and there's "no need to follow up." Do your best to provide an opportunity for the person to receive the validation you intended to provide. If the situation was significant enough to unravel you, chances are that they could still benefit from some support.

RECAP

- Emoting means expressing your genuine reaction to another person's experience.
- You can Emote by doing the following:
  - » Using nonverbal behavior
  - » Stating thoughts that imply emotions
  - » Labeling your feelings using emotion adjectives
- Emoting can be a particularly effective validation skill to use when . . .
  - » They're playing it cool.
  - » You're playing it cool.
- Common Emoting mistakes include the following:
  - » Coming on too strong

> » Striking the wrong chord
> » Losing control

- To *prevent* mistakes, experiment with expressing less intense emotions and refrain from Emoting in crisis situations. If you're worried about controlling your emotions, practice Emoting to validate positive emotions because they're less likely to overwhelm you.

- To *recover* from mistakes, put your emotions aside, attempt a question or two to reengage the person, and try one of the easier validation skills. If you're unable to regain your composure, excuse yourself and follow up with them later.

PRACTICE TIPS

1. Studying audio and visual examples of this skill can help increase your awareness of how to use it effectively. Check out the following audio and visual sources for ideas on where to find people Emoting and practice identifying the modes of expression—nonverbal behavior, implying, labeling—they use. Note: you can engage others in this exercise and make a game out of it. My daughter is nearing the top of the leaderboard in my family; my judgmental cat, on the other hand, has made no progress.

   > » **Television interviews:** Be it primetime or late-night, pay attention to TV hosts conducting guest interviews. These performers have to facilitate conversations with their guests, put them at ease, and quickly establish rapport. As such, the greats—Larry King, Anderson Cooper, etc.—are pros at Emoting.

   > » **Podcasts and radio shows:** Podcasts and radio shows are particularly useful in helping you identify how vocalics (tone, pitch, volume) are used to Emote, because these cues are often more obvious in the absence of other nonverbal behavior. I'd highly

recommend checking out Terry Gross's show, *Fresh Air*. Gross has mastered the art of subtly but clearly Emoting to validate both positive and negative emotions.

» **Television and movies:** Notice when characters Emote to communicate that "they are there, they get it, and they care" about another character's experience, and take particular note of when these exchanges result in your own sense of validation. The films *Good Will Hunting* and Disney's *Inside Out* provide some of the best examples of validation I've ever seen.

2. Try Emoting using nonverbal behavior, implying, and labeling emotions independently this week. You don't have to inhibit the other modes if they arise naturally, but make a concentrated effort to use one of them. If you rarely have conversations that would justify Emoting, you can engineer them by asking a friend, colleague, or acquaintance how they met their partner, what they did after high school, or about any other major life transition. Remember, communication doesn't have to occur in person. Emojis are the modern-day equivalent of nonverbal behavior.

Hint: For *nonverbal behavior*, imagining that the other person is hard of hearing can help you naturally engage nonverbal behavior like facial expressions and gestures. Reminding yourself that less is more can take the pressure off of *implying emotions*. Finally, if *labeling emotions* feels uncomfortable, you can start by stating an emotion as a fact that is not specific to you (e.g., "That is unbelievable" versus "*I* don't believe that" or "How disheartening" versus "*I'm* disheartened to hear that").

CHAPTER 13

DISCLOSE—THE POWER OF ME, TOO

Each one of us has lived through some devastation, some loneliness,
some weather superstorm or spiritual superstorm; when we look at
each other we must say, I understand. I understand how you feel
because I have been there myself.

—MAYA ANGELOU, *RAINBOW IN THE CLOUD*

When I was diagnosed with MS in 2011, I was terrified and completely burnt out by the health-care system. As is often the case with MS, I'd struggled with debilitating symptoms for years and left a slew of specialists in my wake before finally arriving at the cause of my symptoms. I was panicked when I arrived in Washington after our road trip from North Carolina and scheduled an appointment with the first neurologist I could find. He was an older man in a wheelchair who spoke slowly and softly. His lack of an electronic record system gave me pause, as did the dated facade of his office building, but when he disclosed that he, too, suffered from MS, after confirming my diagnosis, I immediately felt like he cared and could empathize with what I was going through. He took a beat to share what he recalled after first being diagnosed and, in so doing, seamlessly validated my experience. I've gone on to work with some of the country's most renowned MS specialists, but I'm not exaggerating when I say that none compare to that quiet man from Seattle, with the paper files and disorganized desk, who took my hand when I started crying and shared his experience with me.

Disclosure, or self-disclosure, entails sharing personal details about yourself that relate to another person's experience or reaction.* As a validation skill, Disclosure demonstrates that you conceptually and emotionally "get it," that you're able to connect with another person's experience, having gone through something similar yourself. At the top of the Validation Ladder, Disclosure brings you face-to-face with the other person, showing them that you see yourself in them and allowing them to see themselves in you. Although not always high risk, self-disclosure often exposes our vulnerabilities, opening us up to potential judgment, rejection, and betrayal. I argue that it's the simple act of taking these risks that allows others to see how much we care.

Disclosure is certainly among the most intimate ways to validate someone, but it doesn't need to be reserved for intimate relationships. Revealing the roots of your empathy is the swiftest and surest way to communicate its depths. And in the light of empathy, qualities like trust and loyalty emerge, providing pathways to deepen or strengthen any relationship.

WHEN LOOSE LIPS SAIL SHIPS

You can use Disclosure to validate someone if you've been in a similar *situation* and can identify with some part of their reaction. For example, you could validate a colleague's concerns about divorcing their life partner by Disclosing that you also went through a divorce and recall having those same concerns at the time. If you haven't been in a similar situation but have experienced and can empathize with another person's *reaction*, Disclosure can still be effective. You might, for example, validate how upset someone

---

* Although Disclosure is not included among the skills in Marsha Linehan's *DBT Manual*, it is listed as a validation skill elsewhere in the DBT literature, where it is also referred to as Reciprocating (Matching) Vulnerability. (Alan E. Fruzzeti and Allison Ruork, "Validation Principles and Practices in Dialectical Behavior Therapy," in *The Oxford Handbook of Dialectical Behaviour Therapy*, ed. Michaela A. Swales [Oxford, UK: Oxford University Press, 2015], 325–44; Fruzzetti and Iverson, "Mindfulness, Acceptance, Validation," 186.)

feels after getting tongue-tied during a high-stakes Zoom meeting by Disclosing that you once cried yourself to sleep after forgetting your lines during a live theater performance.

Like the other skills on the Validation Ladder, Disclosure isn't a tactic used to disarm people. Connecting the dots between someone else's experience and your own is an exercise in empathy. In 2021, Mehmet Ümit Necef, a researcher studying Islamist terrorism, published a paper about an interview he conducted with a jailed terrorist named Enes Ciftci.[1] Early in the interview, Ciftci described an "empty hole inside of me" that he said disappeared once he found Islam. Necef asked Ciftci to elaborate, and as he did, Necef unexpectedly began to reflect on his younger years when he himself identified as a Marxist revolutionary.[2] Ciftci's description of the "empty hole" resonated deeply with Necef, who'd left his family and college to join a violent revolutionary organization during the 1970s in an effort to fill what he described as an "existential emptiness." Necef also had been jailed and interrogated for his activity in the extremist organization.

Early in their discussions, Necef told Ciftci that he did not sympathize with the Islamic State and was against violent groups. He regretted his engagement with leftist extremism but could relate to the experience of becoming radicalized. Necef wrote: "He is talking as I did when I was 18—minus the religious wording."[3] Necef felt an urge to share his history and—despite having some serious concerns about how the Disclosure would play out, including that it might be used against him—he risked it.

His instincts were correct. According to Necef, "My self-disclosure about my engagement with leftist extremism in my youth opened him [Ciftci] up and my clear impression was that he began to trust me." Ciftci wanted to know more about Necef's experience, and the tone of their conversations shifted. "I felt as if the ice between us—the ice between the researcher and the interviewee—was being broken, and our interaction began to take on a rather more relaxed and cordial, in fact more human, character."[4] The Disclosure had a noticeable effect on Ciftci, who began discussing personal issues and problems, all the while referring to Necef either as "elder brother" (*abi*) or "teacher" (*hocam*). As tends to be the case with validation, Ciftci wasn't the only one affected by the Disclosure. In Necef's words:

> Ciftci was no longer my 'research object', somebody whose beliefs
> I did not share in almost all respects. . . . Now he was a human
> being who had chosen a wrong path to realize his political and
> religious ideals, maybe a "lost soul"—just like me in my
> late teens. Gone was the detached researcher, in came the
> ex-extremist, trying to understand a current extremist and
> ending up feeling empathy for a convicted terrorist, whose
> ideology is far removed from where I stand.[5]

I know; I've talked about interviewing terrorists more than once in this book. The reason is because I can think of no other dynamic in which two people are more poised to distrust, dislike, and disagree with each other. Validation's ability to bridge the gap between terrorist and people seeking to stop terrorists is fascinating, specifically because it seems to have a pacifying effect in both directions. So many of the accounts I've combed through read like Necef's—not with either person conceding to the other's beliefs, but with both parties recognizing something of their shared humanity.

DEGREES OF DISCLOSURE

Private medical information, prior history as a violent extremist—my examples so far suggest that Disclosure requires you to share the most intimate details of your life. That's not necessarily the case. Yes, intimate Disclosures tend to be more impactful, but the information you share doesn't have to be top secret or vulnerable for it to be perceived as validating on some level.

When I learn that someone is a vegetarian because of animal welfare concerns like I am, an immediate sense of validation washes over me. I don't have to explain myself or worry that my life choices will cause them to judge me or feel judged by me. I feel accepted and accepting. This degree of validation is similar to what we experience when we realize that someone shares our political beliefs, went to our alma mater, or acknowledges the superiority of the Detroit Pistons above all other basketball teams. Although low-level Disclosures don't consist of emotionally vulnerable information, they still may convey a meaningful amount of validation.

The degree to which a Disclosure is perceived as validating doesn't just depend on the nature of the disclosure; it also depends on the circumstance surrounding it. I can't catalog all of the scenarios in which Disclosure packs a powerful validation punch, but there are two I want to put on your radar because they provide opportunities for some of the deepest forms of connection we're capable of experiencing.

When Disclosure Invalidates Shame

In chapter 8, I talked about the toxicity of shame. Now I want to put my Caroline spin on this topic and discuss how you can use your shame to help others. But first, Brené Brown. No one is more renowned for their work on shame than Brown. She has spent decades researching shame and inspiring conversations about it through her books, podcast, and TED Talk. For the record, getting people to talk about shame is no easy feat. Even if only in the abstract, folks generally don't like to look at, think about, or discuss shame. Our collective avoidance of this topic kinda makes sense, seeing as how our instinct is to respond to feelings of shame by hiding. As Brown puts it, "Shame thrives on secrecy, silence, and judgment."[6]

Talking about shame takes courage. Even when you believe that others should accept you for who you are, if there's a social stigma attached to something you've done or identify with, you risk rejection in talking about it. For instance, I don't feel any shame about having suffered from major depressive disorder. I realize, however, that mental illness has a bit of a stigma attached to it. That's putting it lightly. Mental illness is up there with BO in terms of experiences that are likely to result in people whispering about you behind your back.

When I talk about my history of depression, I risk being judged, misunderstood, and rejected. I have, in my life, been shamed for having this condition, even though I'm not ashamed of it. I do not think I'm unworthy for having suffered from depression, but there are times when I worry others might. Shame experiences include those we're ashamed of and those that might lead us to be shamed by others.

Occasionally, people dare to share their shame experiences with us. They might not say much, sometimes just allude to them, but even subtle nods to shame take guts. If you've experienced something similar to what they describe, you're uniquely positioned to validate them via Disclosure. Disclosing that you can relate to someone's shame experience is empathy at its best. It prioritizes someone's need for acceptance above your fear of being rejected. As a validation skill, Disclosing sends a clear signal that not only do you see and *logically* understand another person's experience, but also that you can *emotionally* understand and relate to what they're going through.

> **DISCLOSING THAT YOU CAN RELATE TO SOMEONE'S SHAME EXPERIENCE IS EMPATHY AT ITS BEST.**

As a result, Disclosing a similar shame experience can end up invalidating the other person's shame. Their connection with you isn't lost; it's deepened. You send the message that "Your truth doesn't drive us apart. It brings us together." This is one of the few exceptions to the "don't invalidate people's emotions" rule. Disclosing that you, too, have done x or identify as y, takes the secrecy, silence, and judgment shame needs to survive out at the knees. It says, "You're safe to talk about that with me. I won't judge you." Put another way, "Your shame is not valid or useful here." Brown defines shame as "the intensely painful feeling or experience of believing that we are flawed and therefore unworthy of love, belonging, and connection."[7] **Invalidating shame through Disclosure validates the other person's worth.**

If you've ever attended an Alcoholics Anonymous (AA) or Narcotics Anonymous (NA) meeting, you might have a sense of how moving it is when folks who understand an experience that most others judge come together to bear witness to it. Shame is contracted through social interactions; that's also how it is healed.

When They Didn't Realize You Could Empathize

In addition to neutralizing another person's shame, validation is uniquely effective at challenging the assumption that "You couldn't possibly understand." When I met with that first neurologist in Seattle, I expected him to be well informed about MS because it's his specialty. I knew his understanding of the disease would be light-years beyond my own and that he'd have firsthand experience in treating it. I did not, however, expect him to be able to relate to what I was going through. The sense of loss, fear, confusion, despair, and pain I was experiencing seemed incomprehensible to someone who hadn't experienced them firsthand. Sure, he could probably guess how I'd respond to the diagnosis after years of breaking this type of news to people, but I didn't expect him to be able to truly empathize with me; his Disclosure, however, proved that he could.

Disclosing that you can relate when someone presumes you can't allows you to swiftly cut through the barriers of their assumptions. It suggests that you're not just one of those people who *thinks* they know what they're talking about; having gone through something similar means you actually might know. As a therapist, I can use all of the other skills on the Validation Ladder to validate a client who is suffering from depression, but there's only one that demonstrates how deeply I see, understand, and empathize with their experience. **Disclosure cuts through the bullshit, grabs them by the shoulders, and says, "I don't judge you; I get it."**

"MY BAD": DISCLOSURE MISTAKES

Just because you can relate to another person's experience doesn't mean you should necessarily start spilling your guts. If Taking

Action is akin to a power tool, Disclosing is like a bomb. It has the power to annihilate people's shame and assumptions. It also can blow up your life if you're not careful. For me, the decision to Disclose or not comes down to effectiveness and tolerance. How confident am I that my disclosure will be *effective* in validating the other person, and can I *tolerate* any judgment or rejection that might arise if it's not? Even if the person I confide in feels validated, I've got to be prepared for them to leak my story on social media or share it with others who might be judgmental or cruel. Again, Disclosures don't always have to be intimate to be validating, but the more private the information is, the more thoughtful you want to be about sharing it.

Even if your Disclosure passes the effectiveness and tolerance test, there are still a bunch of mistakes you can make. I've rounded up the most common errors associated with Disclosure in the following sections, along with my tips on how to avoid and recover from them.

Mistake #1: Overshadowing Their Thing with Your Thing

We've all been exposed to some version of the "Back in my day, I had to walk ten miles in the snow to get to school . . ." comments. Sometimes they're intended to dismiss our emotions or help us "put things in perspective." Every now and then, they represent sincere Disclosure attempts gone sideways. If your experience was more intense or difficult than the other person's, you risk minimizing or even invalidating them. Rather than demonstrating that you understand and can relate to what they're describing, you appear out of touch and self-focused.

> **Solution:** Deference. Highlight what's more exciting, disappointing, or whatever about the other person's experience compared to yours, presuming you can do so authentically. Also, focus more on observations they might share, such as

"Do you find yourself feeling x?" or "I remember thinking y," rather than inadvertently one-upping their thing with yours.

Example: Validating someone who has been experiencing daily nausea for several months.

Thumbs down: "Chronic nausea is the worst. I struggled with it during my last two years of graduate school. I was working on my doctoral dissertation at the time, which I somehow managed to complete. Then I was diagnosed with MS. Nausea turned out to be one of the many symptoms I had to learn to live with."

Thumbs up: "Chronic nausea is the worst. I struggled with it a few years back and found it really debilitating. I can't imagine how you manage the unrelenting desire to puke while raising three kids. Does the smell of food get to you, or are you okay being around it?"

Mistake #2: Losing Focus

Even if you don't overshadow the other person's experience, you could end up getting lost in your story. When we share our experiences, it's natural for people to inquire about them or express an interest in us. That's all fine and good . . . up to a point. If you get caught up in your own story, or the focus of the conversation switches away from the other person for too long, your validation attempt might communicate that you're more interested in sharing your experiences than listening to theirs.

Even if you're not distractible, the conversation can quickly become all about you if the other person interprets your Disclosure as a sign that you want a chance to talk. Conversations are typically a give-and-take, so it's reasonable for someone to misread your Disclosure as an indirect way of saying, "Okay, my turn now." **If the person you're trying to validate tends to focus on the needs**

of others over their own or is highly sensitive, you've got to be extra careful not to let the conversation become about you after Disclosing.

Highly sensitive people are, by definition, sensitive to emotional cues. They also tend to err on the side of attending to others' emotions rather than dismissing them. Faced with an unclear signal (Disclosure) and the desire to meet other people's emotional needs, they'll almost always pivot from talking about themselves to talking about you. And they're freakishly good at it! You'll glance at the clock only to realize you spent the last hour talking about that summer you spent in Italy when your intent was to validate their anxiety about taking an international flight.

Solution: As is the case with Emoting, being intentional about maintaining the focus of the conversation on the person you aim to validate is critical here. Ask questions, use other validation skills, do what got you gotta do—just don't let the topic shift entirely from the other person to you. **Psychologists are told to return the conversation to the client *immediately* after making a Disclosure.** This is another one of those strategies that are buried in articles on psychotherapy, even though it works just as well on blind dates.[8] More than any other, I try to keep the "return it" principle in mind when Disclosing to validate others, especially when my Disclosure has a storytelling quality to it.

Example: Validating a high school senior who is feeling stressed by the college application process.

Thumbs down: "When I was in high school, we had to meet with an academic adviser every week, starting as freshmen, to research schools. Test prep, AP classes, and application writing were all I thought about. Then I got the bright idea to try out for the school play. We were doing *Guys and Dolls* that year, and I thought the play would force me to focus on something other than college. Big mistake. I started . . ."

Thumbs up: "I think the college application process was one of the most stressful periods of my entire life. Did I ever tell you how I fell asleep during the SATs? Yup, I 100 percent passed out. I couldn't sleep the night before the exam because I was afraid I'd sleep through my alarm in the morning. Instead, I ended up being awake for my alarm but falling asleep during the test. How about you? Any sleepless nights so far?"

Mistake #3: Boundary-Crossing

The problem with boundaries is that people talk about them like they're bright, fixed, neon lines that are so obvious they can be seen from outer space. They're not. Boundaries are highly individualized and often difficult to detect. They're determined by a collage of factors, including one's culture, gender, history, and expectations, to name a few. They also change depending on the situation and roles we find ourselves in. Determining someone's boundaries can be like trying to find the three-dimensional image in one of those Magic Eye books from the 1990s: you have to study them closely and squint to find the dimension you're looking for.

When it comes to Disclosing, the specific boundary you're trying to discern is if it's appropriate to open up in response to someone who has opened up to you. Crossing the boundary into inappropriate territory is typically people's greatest fear when it comes to Disclosing, and, I'm not gonna lie, it's a painful line to trip. Boundary-crossing may cause others to question your character and trustworthiness.

Solution: If you are new to this skill, prone to oversharing, or struggle with seeing boundaries, *don't* cannonball into the pool of Disclosure; just dip your toe in. Experiment with low-level Disclosures and gauge the person's response. If you suspect you may have crossed into inappropriate territory, get the hell out of there! Deflect attention away from yourself using the **Mindfulness Skills**, and retreat to a more formal tone while remaining calm and collected. Psychological safety is compromised when boundaries are crossed, but it can be reestablished through steadiness and patience. Like an animal that feels threatened if you approach them too quickly, people need you to step back and stay calm in order to feel safe again.

Mistake #4: Being Too Close to It

If the experience you're thinking about Disclosing is raw, painful, unresolved, or destabilizing for you, keep it to yourself. You might see a once-in-a-lifetime opportunity to validate through Disclosure, but if you're still processing the experience, your attempt at validation is likely to end up burdening the other person. No matter how much you assure someone that "I'm fine," or "I always cry like this," most people are kind at their core and will want to soothe whatever pain they might have inadvertently provoked. If you're too close to it, Disclosing your experience will make it difficult for the other person to talk about theirs.

> **Solution:** Give it space, and play it safe. I don't think I could have Disclosed the emotions I experienced right after my mom was diagnosed with a brain tumor to validate my client, Ella, who lost her mother to cancer. I did, after my mom was in the clear and I'd had space to process the ordeal, but Disclosing any sooner likely would have been a burden to my client and a distraction to me.

If you're not sure you have enough distance to talk about an experience without getting absorbed by it, play it safe and don't Disclose. To be clear, this doesn't mean you shouldn't talk to people about your struggles or pain. For heaven's sake, please do! Just not when your intention is to validate them. **For what it's worth, the degree to which you feel comfortable Disclosing an experience for the purposes of validation can be a subtle indication of how well you've processed it.**

RECAP

- Disclosure entails sharing personal details about yourself that relate to another person's situation or reaction.
- Disclosing less intimate information can be validating, although, when appropriate, intimate Disclosures communicate a greater degree of validation. Disclosing is particularly effective when . . .
  - » Your Disclosure invalidates someone's shame.
  - » They didn't realize how much you get it.
- Disclosure is easy to screw up and can be dangerous if you do. Here are the most common mistakes and how to manage them:

  1. Overshadowing their thing with your thing
  Solution: Disclose with deference, and focus on observations the other person might share rather than the singularity of your experience.

  2. Losing focus
  Solution: Ask questions, use other validation skills, and do what you gotta do to shift the focus back to the other person following your Disclosure.

  3. Boundary-crossing
  Solution: Dip your toe in by experimenting with low-level Disclosures to develop your confidence and familiarity with this skill. If you do cross a boundary, deflect attention away from yourself using the **Mindfulness Skills** and remain calm.

  4. Being *too* close to the experience
  Solution: Give it space, and play it safe.

PRACTICE TIPS

Disclosing is the trickiest validation skill to practice because it's contingent upon other people opening up to you first. That means you'll have to rely more on modeling—observing others Disclosing—to develop this skill. In theory, this should be easy. As the German sociologist Georg Simmel said, "all relations which people have to one another are based on their knowing something about one another."[9] However, just because people disclose on the regular doesn't mean they're always doing it to be validating. You want to become more aware of when Disclosure is used for validation. These are the situations to study, and you'll need a finer comb to find them:

1. As with Emoting, you can look for examples of Disclosing in podcasts and on TV. Reality shows are often chock-full of Disclosing scenes; they're gold to producers who can use them to develop characters and relationships in one fell swoop. Social media is also good for examples of people Disclosing for the purposes of validation, albeit not always successfully. Finally, and most important, reflect on examples from your own life—times when you felt validated by someone's Disclosure or perhaps uncomfortable because of it.

2. Experiment with low-level disclosures. Start to get a feel for sharing details about yourself while swiftly returning the focus of the conversation to the other person. For example, "Love the Pistons hat! I'm a huge fan. Who's your favorite player?" As you get increasingly adept at this skill, experiment with making more vulnerable Disclosures.

PART 3

WHERE CHANGE COMES IN

CHAPTER 14

CH, CH, CH, CHANGES— BEHAVIORAL CHANGE STRATEGIES

The only way to make sense out of change is to plunge into it,
move with it, and join the dance.

—ALAN WATTS, *THE WISDOM OF INSECURITY*

In the summer of 2013, I was locked in a bathroom for a couple of months with a young man who utterly schooled me in behaviorism. Okay, technically, I wasn't locked in there; he was, but I could come and go as needed, which was good because I was pregnant. Also, I should clarify that the young man in question was a feral, three-legged cat I'd rescued from our backyard, now known as Sparrow Baggins.

For the record, I had no intention of spending my summer domesticating a feral cat. When I first spotted him hopping like a bunny in my backyard, scavenging for food, my plan was to catch him and take him to the city's no-kill shelter. I figured they'd fix his broken leg and adopt him out. When I finally trapped and brought him in, the shelter vet took one look at his leg and said it was beyond repair. Sparrow wouldn't survive in the wild with only three legs, she said, and he was too old to domesticate. She told me the only humane option was to euthanize him. If you ask me, this particular shelter was playing it fast and loose with the word *humane*; also, they need to add a giant asterisk next to the "no-kill" description in their title that reads "Unless your kitten is feral and has three legs and we feel like it."

I returned to the front desk to pick up Sparrow, but they refused to release him to me. I wasn't his owner, and my having brought him to the shelter meant he was now in their custody. Yes, this is also the story of how I landed myself in a custody dispute with the state of California. With my pregnant back against the wall, I did what any self-respecting animal lover would do. I lied and said I had an enclosed cat sanctuary attached to my home. By some miracle (or nightmare, if you ask Mat), the lie worked, and Sparrow was released to me. When I got home, I let him loose in our bathroom and locked the door.

By the time Sparrow came into my life, I was already a pro at using behavioral strategies to effect change. I'd completed a doctorate, clinical residency, and postdoc focused on cognitive behavioral therapies, including DBT, and I had studied under some of the field's leading minds. I had a successful clinical practice and a reputation for being able to treat complex behavioral problems. Surely, I could handle a three-legged cat! Or so I told myself as I sat crouched outside the bathroom door, questioning my life choices. In the end, Sparrow proved to be one of my most challenging cases. And as any clinician knows, the harder the case is, the more you stand to learn from it.

Working with Sparrow didn't teach me much about validation per se. Apart from Attending and occasionally Copying his meows so I could pretend we were having meaningful conversations (those were long days), I wasn't exercising my validation skills. When I say I learned a lot from Sparrow, I mean with regard to principles of learning and behaviorism, the so-called change strategies. Our work sharpened my understanding of these techniques and how to apply them.

When it comes to driving specific changes, like encouraging my daughter to clean the garage while I exercise or helping a company reshape a toxic work culture, I think in terms of validation *and* behaviorism. Acceptance *and* change. I attribute most of the success in my career and personal life to this combination of skill sets. Because part 3 is all about how you can combine these approaches to transform your life in ways that matter most to you, I want to quickly review the change strategies, several of which I've mentioned in passing. Folks tend to overestimate the effects of personality and character in determining human behavior, so psychologists often use animals to demonstrate how principles of behaviorism inform change. Rather than deferring to Pavlov's dogs or Skinner's pigeons,* I'm going to rely on my work with Sparrow to explain the various change strategies in this chapter. The remainder of part 3 will look at the intricacies of combining them with validation and applying them to people.

IT'S A MATTER OF CONDITIONING

Classical and operant conditioning are two of the driving forces that determine if, when, and why people (and animals) change their behavior. Both processes rely on the power of association. **Classical conditioning affects involuntary behavior**—after repeatedly pairing the sound of my knocking on the door with food, Sparrow eventually started to twitch his nose and salivate (involuntary responses) at the sound of my knocking on the door. Over time, he began to associate my presence with food, safety, and comfort. Sparrow would go into fight-or-flight mode whenever anyone entered the room, but he'd immediately calm down when he saw it was me. The involuntary heart racing and pupil dilation that comes with sympathetic arousal decreased when he realized it was just mama.

Operant conditioning affects voluntary behavior. Because I was primarily trying to change Sparrow's voluntary behavior—namely hiding, biting, bathroom destruction, etc.—I focused most of my efforts on operant conditioning. Shaping, positive reinforcement, negative reinforcement, extinction, and punishment are the primary tools in the operant conditioning toolbox.

---

* In studying operant conditioning, Skinner famously built a box that would reward the pigeons he placed in it with a food pellet when they pecked a specific key.

When I first brought Sparrow home, I had visions of him curling up to sleep on my chest while I gently stroked his atrophied paw. I knew it was a stretch; I just didn't appreciate how much of a stretch. The first day I risked going into the bathroom, I was horrified to find that my one-armed kitty had managed to shred the wallpaper, tear down the shower curtain, and defile our bathtub. There were shards of glass on the floor from a picture frame he somehow ninjaed off the walls. I had underestimated the "wild" part of "wild animal."

There was no chance in hell Sparrow was going to curl up lovingly in my lap any time soon. I had a lot of shaping ahead of me. **Shaping means reinforcing incremental progress toward a desired behavior.** You look for the teeny-tiniest improvement in someone's current behavior and then reinforce it.

Sparrow's MO at the time was to bolt behind the toilet when I entered the room and stay hidden until I left. I figured a slight improvement would be if he took one small hop-step out of his hiding spot, so I began the shaping process by placing some tasty wet food (reward) about six inches from where he was hiding. I'd then sit at the opposite end of the bathroom and wait up to two hours for him to take the bait. If he didn't come out, I'd leave with the wet food and he'd have to wait a few hours for some less desirable dry food to be dispensed from an automatic feeder. Initially, he ignored me (I'll explain why in a moment); then, one day, he decided to risk his life for a taste of whatever it was that smelled so good. And he quickly realized it was *worth it*! After a week or two, Sparrow was coming out within seconds of me placing the food down.

Having conditioned Sparrow to take one step out from his hiding place for food, I then moved the bowl out another six inches. Little man was not pleased with my games. He waited more than an hour to come out the first day I made this change, but by the end of the week, he was again doing his cute little bunny hops toward the food within minutes of my placing it down. We progressed sequentially in this way: I moved the food closer and closer to me over time until he eventually had to crawl into my lap to get it and tolerate me lifting him off the ground while he ate. Within several months, I had a sweet, three-legged cat resting on my chest while I gently stroked his atrophied paw. Such is the power of shaping.

In my work with Sparrow, I initially relied on food to *positively reinforce* his behavior of coming toward me. I talked briefly about positive reinforcement in chapter 2, where I defined it as a reward given *after* a behavior occurs, which increases the likelihood that the behavior will be repeated. Now that we're looking at actually applying these principles, I want to highlight one of the biggest mistakes people make in trying to reinforce others: they confuse *rewards* with *reinforcements*. **For a reward to be considered a reinforcement, it needs to affect behavior.**

I mentioned that Sparrow initially showed no interest in coming out for the food, which was wet as opposed to dry and came in a can with the image of a cat wearing pearls on the side of it. Cats prefer wet food to dry, and the pearls led me to believe I'd purchased a delectable delicacy. But Sparrow wasn't having it. After several failed attempts to lure him out from hiding with the cat-pearl-brand stuff, I turned to Reddit and found a thread about how Gerber's chicken-flavored baby food is irresistible to cats. Not joking—it's known as "kitty crack" in cat socializing circles. I bought a jar, took it into the bathroom when Sparrow was good and hungry, and BOOM, we were in business! Before, with the wet food, I'd spent hours waiting for him to move, only to have him run out the clock on me, but after just twenty minutes of that wafting chicken baby-food smell, he caved. The food I tried initially was a reward. He liked it but not enough to change his behavior. Gerber's chicken-flavored baby food was a reinforcement.

Negative reinforcement is not what you think. By that, I mean it's not punishment. The "negative" in negative reinforcement does this term a real disservice. **Despite being "negative," negative reinforcement feels *good* to the individual receiving it because it takes away something aversive or undesirable.** When people ran out of the room after Sparrow lunged and hissed, he was negatively reinforced for lunging and hissing. His behavior resulted in aversive humans leaving him the hell alone, which made him more likely to do it.

One of my earliest tasks was to *extinguish* Sparrow's aggressive behavior by ignoring it (with the help of multiple layers of protective clothing). **Rather than providing reinforcements for desired behavior, extinction reduces problematic behavior by eliminating the reinforcements that are maintaining it.**

Finally, punishment is an aversive consequence for a behavior. Traveling animal circuses are a testament to the fact that you can rely largely on punishment to change behavior. But if you care about the well-being of the other person or your relationship with them, punishments should be mild and used sparingly. Alan Kazdin, PhD, is a brilliant behaviorist renowned for his work with oppositional children. In grad school, I was trained in his method, parent management training, which is used to help parents manage various behavioral problems in children.[1] One of the points Kazdin makes is that punishing kids teaches them what not to do, but it doesn't show them what to do. Kazdin's words were at the front of my mind when working with Sparrow. Without severe punishments like starving or hurting him, I couldn't draw out the behavior I wanted. He did not understand what I expected him to do, much less have any incentive to do it. It took a combination of shaping and extinction for Sparrow to make the desired changes. Once he'd made significant progress, I might punish regressions by removing food or leaving the room. **But growth was always achieved through reinforcing progress and withholding the reinforcements driving problematic behavior.**

I used to reflect on the teachings of Kazdin and my experience with Sparrow when Havana threw tantrums as a young kid. It seemed obvious that she should know what to do—stop yelling and throwing shit. But just like Sparrow, she had to learn how to do that. She needed to be reinforced for taking a time-out, deep breathing, distracting herself, or calming herself down. Yes, she knew we wanted her to stop screaming at the top of her lungs, but she hadn't yet learned how to regulate her emotions. In addition to reinforcing progress toward emotion regulation, I needed to be careful not to reinforce tantrum behavior with attention. Note that even negative attention—say, through yelling or disagreeing with someone—can still be reinforcing. As a dear colleague of mine used to say, "Don't reinforce arguing with arguing."

Before we wrap up this section, I need to warn you that in the land of modern-day behaviorism, the term *behavior* is used loosely and includes everything from thoughts to emotions to sweating. This broader definition of behavior is significant because it implies that a person's thoughts and feelings can be shaped, much like an animal's behavior. Although I knew that principles of behaviorism are not limited to observable behavior, it ironically took socializing a three-legged cat for me to realize how critical they are to changing the complicated dynamics and expectations that define human relationships.

In my work with Sparrow, I saw that he learned to *like* me through operant and classical conditioning. As his behavior changed in response to our work, so did his emotions. Suspicion transitioned into trust. Fear and distress morphed into affinity and fondness. I began to see how my relationships with people had been shaped in much the same way—not through the unknowable inner workings of the big black box between our earholes but through the basic principles of behaviorism that affect thoughts and emotions as much as they do behaviors. In my defense, I think the "behavior" in behaviorism was subconsciously throwing me off. It should really be called "changeism," but I suspect spell-check has gotten in the way of us updating the lexicon.

Post Sparrow, I fully embraced the notion that people's inner experiences can be shaped just like their behavior. When I encountered resistance, I stopped assuming that people are too complex (I can't get a narcissist to show remorse, I can't help someone who blames everyone else for their problems, etc.) and, instead, focused on my methods (I need a different type of "food"). I also adopted the ever-so-dialectical mantra that "People are complicated *and* governed by basic principles of change." Through this lens, I came to appreciate that although people respond to basic rewards like food, the inter- and intrapersonal changes they make are usually dictated by more complex reinforcements and punishments—namely, validation and invalidation. People need emotional validation to thrive and, in some cases, survive. The need for validation, just like the need for food, makes it a potent reward that may be powerful enough to operate as a reinforcement. This need also explains why emotional invalidation, just like food deprivation, should never be used intentionally to punish someone.*

MODELING AND PROBLEM-SOLVING

Modeling and problem-solving are two other change strategies, although they're associated more with learning theory than with traditional behaviorism. I mentioned modeling in chapter 5 in explaining why I use media examples to illustrate various validation skills. The takeaway is that we learn through observation—this goes for complex behaviors like validation and more basic skills like how to jump high enough to reach a particular food source.** Modeling, like principles of behaviorism, applies to *thoughts, emotions,* and *behaviors.* Self-doubt, body dysmorphia, and feelings of entitlement can all be "taught" through modeling. The upside is that self-validation and gratitude also can be learned in much the same way.

---

* If you're worried about all the people you've unintentionally tortured with emotional invalidation through the years, you can relax. We all experience and communicate invalidation from time to time, just like we all experience hunger and thirst. It's part of life. Invalidation becomes problematic when it is severe, pervasive, or used intentionally to punish someone.

** Side story: My older cat, Elmo, always jumped straight up onto the kitchen counters because she required no special accommodations to reach them. After Sparrow came along, Elmo started jumping from the floor to some lower shelves and *then* to the counter. Three-legged Sparrow was able to follow her example and soon found himself on top of the kitchen counters, where he discovered, THERE'S SO MUCH MORE FOOD! Curiously, Elmo abandoned the lower shelf method after Sparrow had mastered it, reverting to the more efficient floor-to-counter approach. Elmo earned a Good Samaritan badge for her assistance with Sparrow, but she refuses to wear her Girl Scout sash, which I think we can all agree is a real shame.

Problem-solving, as you know, is the process of finding solutions to problems. Once again, the term *problem* is used broadly by psychologists and includes everything from a person's emotions (e.g., I want to be less irritable) to logistical issues (e.g., I need to find a place to put the feral animal I brought home).

The ever-critical "solving" component of problem-solving entails techniques like brainstorming, skills training, and experimentation. These concepts are common enough, so I'll leave it at that. Sorry, no cute stories about how I helped Sparrow solve his problems with his sister, Mindee McMinderstein. He's a cat, and even change strategies have their limits.

MOVING FORWARD

In the final four chapters, I'll discuss my tips on combining the validation skills from part 2 with the change strategies in this chapter. As you begin thinking about how to apply what you've learned, there are some lessons from Sparrow I hope you'll keep in mind. The first is that behaviorism doesn't apply only to behavior. Increasing intimacy, learning to accept yourself, and improving a team's culture, for instance, all constitute meaningful changes that abide by the principles of behaviorism.

Second, validation is like food. Every single person wants to feel accepted and seen. Period. **If someone doesn't respond positively to validation, it's because you haven't actually validated them.** Just as you wouldn't doubt that an animal needs food, don't question a person's need for validation, and don't judge yourself for desiring it.*

Third, just because you succeed at validating someone doesn't mean they'll necessarily change how and when you want them to. For one thing, many of the positive changes associated with validation—increased trust, intimacy, etc.—require time and

---

* If you're still struggling with the idea that it's okay to desire external validation, try replacing the term *validation* with *acceptance* or any of the other defining features of validation (i.e., *mindfulness, understanding,* or *empathy*).

consistency. For another, you're not God. Even if you combine validation with the strategies in this chapter, stronger associations, reinforcements, punishments, skill deficits, or sources of influence in a person's environment can undermine your efforts. Expect this. Count on it. Rather than blaming the individual or writing them off as incapable of change, study the circumstances, including any constraints. Accept the conditions and then change your approach. If and when that fails, remember that the relationship between acceptance and change is bidirectional. You may need to accept that some conditions are beyond your control, but the acceptance itself will culminate in change—perhaps not the specific change you seek or the degree to which you want it, but I've learned never to underestimate the power of acceptance or the effect it can have on one's life.

Finally, a word about manipulation: when Skinner's technology of behavior* began making waves in the 1960s and 1970s, there was an outrage of concern over how people might use it to manipulate and control others. These days, I think most of us see technologies like artificial intelligence (AI) as a greater threat to the enslavement of the human race, but I still want to address the behaviorism = manipulation concern as it pertains to validation because it comes up from time to time. When it does, I reiterate that validation is the *authentic* communication of acceptance. Misleading and deceiving people are incompatible with validation and will only hurt your relationships. I also add that if a person's only motivation for accepting others is so they can exploit them, they're going about it all wrong. Anyone who puts the work into cultivating mindfulness, understanding, and empathy will be changed in the process, and not in ways that are a disservice to the person they're trying to "manipulate." I, for one, wish more people would try to manipulate me with acceptance and validation.

---

* Behaviorism is often referred to as the "technology of behavior." In modern-day cognitive behavioral approaches, it's also known as the "technology of change."

CHAPTER 15

RAISING EMOTIONALLY INTELLIGENT CHILDREN— VALIDATION AND PARENTING

I still hear you humming Mama. . . . The color of your words saying, "Let her
be. She got a right to be different. She gonna stumble on herself one of these
days. Just let the child be." And I be Mama.

—SONIA SANCHEZ, "DEAR MAMA," *SHAKE LOOSE MY SKIN*

As you might imagine, there are meaningful differences in what it takes to be effective with your kid versus your boss versus yourself. The validation skills and change strategies are consistent across the board; insights into how to apply them in different types of relationships are what we turn to now. This chapter covers parent-child dynamics. I'll discuss how to use validation to reinforce kids for being awesome and how to discipline kids without scarring them for life. The next two chapters look at intimate and professional relationships with adults, and the last focuses on the easiest relationship to overlook: the one you have with yourself. If you don't interact much with other adults, never plan on being around kids, or transcended your sense of self on a recent ayahuasca trip, I still recommend reading the chapters on these topics. They reinforce the concepts in this book, and I promise there's something in them for everybody.

VALIDATION AS REINFORCEMENT:
FINDING THE GOLDEN SNITCH

I once worked with a client, Keith, who wanted to get better at Emoting to validate his wife. So for homework one week, I asked him to look for opportunities to practice Emoting with others. I should note that I'd already taught Keith about behaviorism and discussed how validation can be reinforcing, but he hadn't experienced these effects firsthand.

A few days after our session, Keith's wife and nine-year-old daughter had a fight that ended with their kiddo being sent to her room. After a while, Keith went in to check on his daughter, at which point she yelled, "I know! I know I'm not doing this right, and I'm trying to do it better . . ." before launching into one of those artfully crafted diatribes kids can construct on the fly when they're mad at one of their parents. Keith sat there listening, neither stoking the flames nor trying to put them out, while his daughter vented about how totally and stupidly unfair Mom was being. As Keith Attended, he began to focus on what he was feeling. And then, just like that [fingers snapped for effect], he saw an opportunity to knock out his validation homework *and* test his therapist's theory that validation can be reinforcing. He waited a little longer and then interjected, "Can I change the subject? I know you're mad right now, but all I can think about is how you came out and said, 'I'm really trying to do this better.'" His daughter looked at him like, "Is this a test?" Keith continued, "I don't have the courage to say things like that or even admit them to myself. I'm so proud of you [labeled emotion] and impressed [labeled emotion]. I am glad [labeled emotion] to be your dad so that I can learn from you." And with that, Keith started to tear up (nonverbal expression of emotion from a dude who is not one to cry).

Then, in what felt like a scene plucked from a 1980s sitcom, Keith's daughter left the room and apologized to her mom. And not with one of those lame *sor-ryyyyy*s said through gritted teeth, but a heartfelt, validating apology complete with a hug and ideas on what she could do next time to keep things from escalating.

Kiddo's reaction was *impressive*, but I want to focus on the remarkable response from Keith that preceded it. I mean, can you imagine how it would have felt, as a kid, to have your dad zoom in on what you did well when you were expecting him to focus on what you'd done wrong? Much less have him tell you, with tears in his eyes, that he's proud to be your father? I can't personally relate to that experience, but I imagine it's one I wouldn't soon forget. And that's the point. People encode the relationship between what they did and how it made them feel. Behaviors that result in strong positive emotions are likely to be repeated: the kid reinforced for acknowledging their role in a conflict is more likely to do so in the future—perhaps in as little as ten minutes, but don't hold me to that. The validation you give a child doesn't need to be as dramatic as it was in this example, but it must resonate deeply with them to be reinforcing. **Over the years, I've found that Proposing, Emoting, and Disclosing tend to be the most reinforcing validation skills to use with kiddos and teens.** I should note that although validation is a great way to reinforce kids, you should not use it solely for this purpose. Validation, like love, must never be withheld. It should be abundant in a child's environment *and* used intentionally to reinforce behavior.

One of the many obstacles we parents face is that it's hard for us to see the progress, growth, and maturity our kids demonstrate over time, partly because we're always around them. But also because, let's face it, the statement "I know I'm not doing this right" isn't nearly as salient as the screaming that came before it or the spiteful complaining that followed. Identifying something to reinforce with validation as a parent is like trying to spot the Golden Snitch if you're Harry Potter—you've got to ignore all the other shit that's being thrown at you and focus intently on finding a flitting ball of light that will disappear the instant you take your eye off it.

There is always a Golden Snitch to be found, and by that I mean some slightly better or less offensive behavior to reinforce with validation. I keep this in mind as a parent and when working with young people who have severe behavioral problems. Sometimes I can't see the Snitch through the fog of my expectations or the dust a kid kicks up as they spin out, but I always trust that it will appear. If I work with them long enough and look hard enough, eventually, I'll spot it.

Fortunately, most opportunities to reinforce kids with validation occur outside of conflicts. Although it's easier to authentically validate someone if you're not physically restraining them from hurting you, you'll still need to keep a keen eye out for that elusive Golden Snitch—the opportunity to reinforce desired behavior with validation—to spot it. An average Quidditch game lasts only an hour or two; parenting is a 24/7 gig. What follows is an example of a near miss by none other than the person writing this book. You'll probably spot the Snitch immediately, proving my point that this shit isn't as apparent when it's your kid.

Havana's previous school graciously provided the students with a morning snack. Except, it wasn't a snack so much as a dessert packed with just enough sugar and calories to ruin Havana's appetite for lunch, leaving her ravenous by three p.m. After discussing this problem with her, she agreed that she should skip the morning snack. So that's what she did. I'm sorry; I should have said that's what she *tried* to do. Pastries shrink-wrapped in plastic are Havana's version of Sparrow's Gerber chicken-flavored baby food. The smell of cellophane and sugar is enough to force her to go against her better judgment and, if it came down to it, probably risk her life. We needed a better plan. I soon realized the solution was obvious: "If you have the treat at school," I told her, "then you can't have dessert after dinner." She LIVES for her post-dinner treats, so although she was not a fan of this plan, she couldn't deny that it would probably work. But it didn't. Each day the following week, I asked if she resisted the morning treat. Each and every time, the response was a big, fat "Nope." By the fifth straight day of this, I was frustrated, disappointed, and annoyed. Then, out of the corner of my eye, I spotted a Golden Snitch. I went for it.

"You didn't lie once this week." Havana eyed me suspiciously from across the dinner table. Seriously, why do kids always think we're sus when we try to validate them?! "You could have said you skipped the morning snack so you could get dessert after dinner, but you didn't. Not once. It must have been upsetting to lose your dessert and disappoint me [Proposing], but you still did the right thing. I'm so freaking proud of you, babe [Emoting]." Havana came over and wrapped her arms around me. "It was! It was hard for me!" she exclaimed.

Havana was at an age when she was experimenting with lying. She was a lousy liar, so we usually caught her, but she was beginning to see that it was an obvious solution to many of a kid's problems. Her lying wasn't egregious or frequent; it was just low level enough that any improvement was easy to overlook, as I almost did. After that, I kept an eye out for Golden Snitch opportunities to reinforce honesty with validation. I caught a couple, and with each, the incidents of lying became fewer and farther between. When asked to describe herself in three words for an "About Me" project the following year, Havana chose *silly, creative,* and *honest.* Not only did she come to see herself as an honest person and behave accordingly, this quality also became a point of pride for her.

Catching the Golden Snitch requires vigilance, and there's a bit of a learning curve, but I've got some tips to help quickly advance your game:

- Any time a kid is struggling to make progress in one domain (e.g., skipping the morning snack), look to see if there's progress in another (e.g., honesty). Kids do not develop when and where we expect them to. **Ask yourself, "If I had to reinforce something, what would it be?"**

- **Be on the lookout for small signs of growth, and remember the principle of *shaping.*** With kids, progress can look like having a tantrum without throwing anything (presuming they were previously doing both), yelling but not swearing, or initiating a chore without completing it (again, assuming this is progress).

- **Focus on a child's efforts, intentions, and character.** If a kid shows you a poorly drawn picture, you might not see much to reinforce, much less authentically validate. If instead, you reflect on the amount of time, patience, and perseverance they demonstrated while working on it, you'll find many of the qualities you want them to develop. Reinforcing kids with validation isn't about ensuring everyone gets a trophy; it's about prioritizing process over product and progress over perfection. *Note: if your kid produced a shit drawing and didn't put much time or effort into it, don't worry about reinforcing them. You can be nice and accept the drawing graciously, but if you don't see a behavior you want to increase, you don't need a reinforcement-caliber response.*

Perhaps the best thing you can do to increase your odds of finding opportunities to reinforce your kid with validation is to keep the intention top of mind. Change your phone's wallpaper to a picture of the words *Reinforcement and validation,* add them to your daily calendar, or find another way to cue yourself to reflect on these concepts. That was all Keith had to guide him. He'd learned the basic principles of behaviorism and was making a concerted effort to practice Emoting. Now he's in the running for next year's Gryffindor captain.

Punishment—Managing Problems Without Creating Them

When I bring up the topic of punishment, parents act like I've broken out a joint for us to share in the school bathroom. They get all giddy with nervous excitement and go on high alert like they're expecting to be busted at any moment. I get it. *Punishment* has become something of a bad word in parenting circles. Therapists are trained to underemphasize it in their work with parents, sometimes discussing the concept only after months of drilling positive reinforcement. Decreasing the emphasis on punishment with parents is important because most tend to overuse it. Big time. Cases of actual abuse aside, many parents are too frequent, severe, and unpredictable with punishment for it to be effective.[1]

That said, of course, there need to be consequences for problematic behavior! I could refer to all of the parenting research that substantiates this point, but I don't need to because if you've spent any time around kids, then you know that they're like little *Jurassic Park* dinosaurs who will destroy the park and probably kill you when they realize the fence is off. Consequences, punishments, contingencies—whatever you call them—are important. Period. The question isn't whether or not you use them; it's *how* you use them.

I can't cover all the dos and don'ts of punishment, but there is one point I want to spend a beat on: emotional invalidation. It's all too easy to invalidate a child's emotions when they are acting out of control, but this insidious and overlooked form of punishment hurts far more than it helps. There is a boatload of research on the negative effects of invalidating children's emotions during conflicts, so I'll just stick to the highlights:

- Emotional invalidation during parent-child conflicts is highly correlated with anger, oppositional defiance, and externalizing problems in adolescents.[2]
  Translation: Invalidation pisses off teens and may lead them to act out.

- Children are more likely to become dysregulated when parents invalidate their emotions during conflicts; they're also more likely to develop maladaptive coping strategies associated with mental health problems.[3]

Translation: Parents who invalidate their children have children who invalidate themselves.

- There is a strong association between emotional invalidation during parent-child conflicts and subsequent self-harm in adolescents.[4]
  Translation: None needed.

Okay, so, nasty stuff. The importance of punishment, alongside the harmful effects of emotional invalidation, begs the question: how do you discipline your children without invalidating them? To answer this question, I'll refer you to the bylaws of validation from chapter 3, which clearly state that you should only **validate the valid** and that **emotions are always valid**, at least as far as you're concerned.

Children often behave in ways that are problematic in terms of the rules, the law, and, you know, basic survival. It's important to invalidate problematic *behavior* in children. That's called parenting. What you want to avoid invalidating is kids' *emotions*. The studies I mentioned spoke to the effects of emotional invalidation on children. The line between invalidating a kid's behaviors and invalidating their emotions is easy to overlook but devastating to cross.

To stay on the right side of that line when disciplining children, focus on their behavior, not their character or feelings. Let a mild punishment—a temporary loss of a privilege, a short time-out, extra chores—do the work. When providing feedback, focus on what the child did (observable behavior), and be specific.

Feedback	Invalidation
I know you're excited, but it's not okay to barge into the bathroom when I'm peeing to ask if you can play at Sophie's house.	Get out of here! You never think about others.
I'm disappointed you didn't turn in your writing assignment.	You don't take school seriously.
It's okay to be sad and upset; it's not okay to scream.	This isn't something to cry about!

Ideally, you can validate a kid's emotions while also providing feedback on their behavior (e.g., it's okay to be *sad* and *upset*; it's not okay to scream), but that's not always possible. When parents ask me how to validate a kid who is working themselves up, my answer is, "Don't." If your kiddo falls dramatically during a tantrum and then wails as though they've been mortally injured, or looks in the mirror when crying only to cry harder, attention and validation are likely to further dysregulate them.[5] That said, it's important to recognize that their feelings are valid. Yes, they're behaving in ways that will make them feel worse, but they are genuinely dysregulated. Oddly enough, their urge to heighten negative emotions is valid, too, in a way.

Ever croon aloud to REM's "Everybody Hurts" in the shower after a hard day? No? Maybe something more recent than "Everybody Hurts" but similarly heart-wrenching? No? Okay, maybe I'm the only one who feels inexplicably compelled to draw out negative emotions even when I know it will make me more upset. Except, I know I'm not because "Everybody Hurts" sold like a zillion copies, and nobody listens to that song to feel better. The point is that human beings are bizarrely wired to amplify negative emotions. When we're mad, we want to rant and rave, not meditate or watch videos of soldiers being reunited with their dogs on YouTube. When we're sad, we isolate ourselves, turn off the lights, and listen to "Everybody Hurts." Sometimes, this tendency to act on emotions becomes a full-blown disorder, but we all do it to some degree.

Although the urge to heighten negative emotions is valid in that it's normal, *acting* on that urge is not effective or helpful to a kiddo who's tantruming. A child imploding before your eyes is in a heightened state of sympathetic arousal—their lizard brains have taken over, which means their already limited capacity for higher reasoning has been reduced to zero. Focusing your attention, be it positive or negative, on problematic behavior can reinforce it, so your best move is to ignore the flailing, facilitate self-soothing if your kiddo is open to it, or distract them by whatever means possible. Rather than focusing on validation, in these moments, you just

INVALIDATING COMMENTS SAID IN ANGER TO A CHILD OFTEN BECOME THE NEGATIVE SELF-TALK THAT HAUNTS THEM INTO ADULTHOOD.

need to be careful not to invalidate your child's emotions. Statements like, "What's wrong with you?!" or "I don't care if you hurt yourself" or "You're too old for this" are easy to let slip when things are chaotic, but these words are not soon forgotten. On the contrary, the hurt they cause makes them stand out in a kid's memory. Invalidating comments said in anger to a child often become the negative self-talk that haunts them into adulthood.

DISCIPLINE VERSUS CONFLICT RESOLUTION

You might need to ignore tantrums or use mild punishments to address behavioral issues, but these strategies are insufficient to resolve conflicts with children. Confusing discipline with conflict resolution has led to the ever-pervasive "pretend nothing happened" approach to parenting, which goes something like this: Kiddo is given a time-out or sent to their room. After a short time, or after the child has calmed down, they can return to the tribe. Everything then goes back to normal as though nothing happened. If apologies are offered, they're said quickly or in passing. This approach isn't abusive by any means, but it is woefully incomplete. Rather than being reinforced for regulating themselves, the child's success is ignored. Instead of having valid emotions acknowledged, they're dismissed. When conflicts are consistently "resolved" in this manner, kids don't develop the skills to process their feelings and correct for mistakes; they learn only to move on and pretend nothing happened.

For discipline to rise to the bar of conflict *resolution*, it must be followed by a *debrief*. Debriefs are when emotional validation, repairs, and reinforcement can occur. These conversations should be gentle and happen *after* the storm has passed and everyone has calmed down. In my experience, bedsheet forts and dark rooms with warm covers create the perfect vibe for debriefs. As for structuring the conversation, I use a "what happened for you" approach in which each person takes turns describing what they observed, thought, and felt during the conflict while the other person looks for something to validate.*

I always let the kiddo go first, presuming they want to. This little gesture offers them a sense of control after having recently lost it. If you use my approach, be prepared for your kid to wildly mischaracterize you and the situation in describing their perspective. If this "what happened for you" thing ever catches on, I want to commission an illustrator to draw the scenes kids describe in these conversations so we can turn their depictions into a graphic novel. It would be both terrifying and hilarious. I imagine our kids would say the same about our versions of the conflict, but kids can't afford illustrators or commission graphic novels, so I don't think we have anything to worry about.

Orienting kids toward expressing what they were *thinking* and *feeling* during the conflict—as opposed to what you, the parent, were doing to provoke them—is one way to keep these debriefs from derailing into "he said, she said" debacles. Biting your lip and using your **Mindfulness Skills** also will help. If you do correct a child's narrative—because it's just so off base, how could you not?!—try to take an "I can see how it could have seemed that way" angle. For example: "Hon, I didn't throw a basketball at you. I was driving on the highway, and there weren't any basketballs in the car. I can see, though, how my tone and words might have felt like a lot hitting you all at once. Did you feel like I was throwing a lot of hurt at you?"

Although you might disagree with some of the dramatic details your kiddo describes, you always want to try to identify and validate the child's emotions. "It *hurts* to feel like someone isn't

---

* If you noticed that my "what happened for you" approach is similar to the Gottman-Rapoport Intervention technique I described in chapter 7, then you, footnote reader, have impressed me once again!

listening to you, especially when it's your dad," or "I'd be *frustrated*, too, if I had to share a new toy with my sister." Debriefs are all about teaching children how to recognize and validate their feelings. Just because they were ineffective in managing them doesn't mean the emotions they experienced were bad or wrong. **It might be appropriate for a child to feel guilty for acting out, but we never want them to feel ashamed of who they are or how they feel.**

In addition to providing emotional validation, **look for opportunities to apologize** for any regrettable things you said or did during the conflict. And none of this "I'm sorry you felt that way" business. Apologies should clearly describe what you did wrong, include the words *I'm sorry*, and end with thoughts on how you'll repair the relationship or change your behavior. If you can validate your emotions while taking responsibility for your behavior, you're really kicking butt. For example: "I raised my voice more than I should have. I'm sorry for that. It's okay to feel *angry*; it's not okay to yell. Next time, I'll take a time-out when I start feeling that way." Remember, if you want your kids to take responsibility for their mistakes, you need to model how it's done.

After your kiddo has shared their perspective and you've validated their emotions, *then* it's time to share "what happened for you." Make a point to express what you were *thinking* and how you *felt* during the conflict. Try to identify emotions beyond frustration, annoyance, or other shades of anger. Your kid—and possibly the neighbors—already knows you were angry. You can mention it, fine, but try to paint yourself as more than just a cartoon character with steam coming out of their ears. Examples include the following:

"I was *afraid* someone was going to get hurt."
"I was *disappointed* in myself for not knowing how to help you."
"I was *confused* by your frustration."

Finally, encourage your kids to validate you by asking them questions like, "Does that make sense?" "Have you ever felt that way?" "Can you see how I got there?" Having just modeled validation in your conversation with them, this is as good a time as any to help them practice it. You don't need to force the issue if they refuse to engage. This exercise is less about getting you the validation you deserve, and more about providing the scaffolding for kids to develop the skills they need.

TAKEAWAYS FOR REFRIGERATORS

I'm a "put it on the refrigerator so I don't forget" type of parent, so I wanted to conclude this chapter with points that could easily be printed and taped to your appliance of choice.

- Validation should be abundant in a child's life *and* used intentionally to reinforce them for being awesome.
- To find those elusive Golden Snitch opportunities to reinforce good behavior with validation:
  - » Look for *small* signs of growth, and remember the principle of *shaping*.
  - » Focus on a child's efforts and intentions.
  - » Ask yourself, "If I had to reinforce something, what would it be?"
- When disciplining children, don't compound punishments with emotional invalidation. Keep feedback specific to the child's observable behavior, and validate their emotions whenever possible.
- Debrief with kiddos after big arguments to validate their emotions, catch Golden Snitches, and model apologies.
- Use the "what happened for you" approach to keep debriefs on track, and consider commissioning an artist to capture the "precious moments" you and your children describe.

CHAPTER 16

THE UNIVERSAL LOVE LANGUAGE—VALIDATION IN INTIMATE RELATIONSHIPS

I felt it shelter to speak to you.

—EMILY DICKINSON, IN A LETTER TO THOMAS WENTWORTH HIGGINSON, 1878

Note: this chapter does *not* speak to relationships involving intimate partner violence. As I said in chapter 8, a victim of abuse is not in a position to change their abuser's behavior.

TRAINING YOUR PARTNER

Most parents already think about rewards and punishments with their kids, so when I tell my Sparrow stories and focus on behavioral concepts with parents, they nod along knowingly. When I introduce this material to couples, however, I'm met with looks of alarm and the occasional, "Did you just compare my wife to a three-legged cat?" Yes, I did, but that's not the point. The point is that principles of change affect all of our relationships equally, whether we're aware of them or not. It might be unsettling to think that you should approach getting your partner to cook with you in the same way you would go about domesticating a feral cat, but here we are. Ignoring principles of change doesn't make them go away; it just increases the chance that they'll work against you. In intimate relationships, the principle we're most punished for over-looking is punishment.

Parents are mindful of punishment with kids because they use it intentionally and talk about it openly: "You're gonna get a time-out" or "She should lose screen time if she doesn't finish her homework." In intimate relationships, punishments tend to be in-conspicuous and are often unintentional. You may not have meant to punish your partner for doing the grocery shopping imperfectly, but when you discovered they forgot the milk and rolled your eyes, that's exactly what happened. The insidious nature of punishment allows it to build up like an undetected carbon monoxide leak that slowly loosens each partner's grip on reality. And yet, somehow, I'm the ridiculous one for talking about reinforcement, punish-ment, and three-legged cats when they come to see me for help. Go figure.

Thanks to our old friend/devil on everyone's shoulder, the negativity bias, we tend to over-index on negative aspects of our relationships while paying less attention to the good stuff. The neg-ativity bias is particularly problematic in long-term relationships, in which anger, frustration, and resentment can build up over time around issues like how one's partner spends money, approaches parenting, or refuses to even consider watching season 1 of *Eupho-ria*. If enough negativity accumulates, one or both partners might find themselves in what marriage experts call negative sentiment override (NSO).[1] A person in NSO perceives their partner's state-ments, attitudes, and behaviors negatively, even when they're ob-jectively neutral or positive. For example, rather than giving their hubby the benefit of the doubt when he doesn't respond immedi-ately to a text message, someone in NSO might entertain thoughts like, "He is trying to prove his time is more important than mine. What type of person doesn't have the decency to respond to his wife?!" NSO can make us more inclined to punish our partners for what we don't like rather than reinforce them for what we appreci-ate. The downstream effects of these biases are problematic be-cause, as I've said before, if you care about the well-being of the other person or your relationship with them, punishments should be mild and used sparingly.

Two additional issues in romantic relationships can cause them to become petri dishes for punishment. First, we seem hardwired to disregard the principle of shaping when it comes to the people we sleep with. It's worse than that. Instead of reinforcing progress in our partners, we tend to punish it with invalidation. Here are some examples from couples I've worked with:

Example #1

Chris and Jordan want to feel more supported by each other. For Chris, this means having Jordan help out more around the house. Jordan makes an effort by doing the laundry but forgets to put the clothes in the dryer. Chris realizes wet clothes are sitting in the washer and flips their shit.

Example #2

Both partners agree that sex is a problem. Marcia wants to increase sexual intimacy, but Clara feels overwhelmed by this request. Clara invites Marcia to take a bubble bath. They don't have sex, but the bath is sensual and a big step for Clara. In their next couples therapy session, Marcia wants to discuss why they didn't have sex.

Example #3

Juanita and John both want John to be more involved with the kids. Juanita specifically wants John to take a more active role in managing parenting responsibilities. John decides to take the kids shopping for back-to-school supplies. Juanita thanks John afterward but then returns everything he bought because she found way better prices at Target.

In that last example, it might seem like Juanita rewarded John by saying "thank you." On its own, her thank you was well and good, but returning the items discredited John's attempt and undermined his competence. Juanita's oversight speaks to my second point—we tend to underestimate what registers as punishing to our partners. Although the effect was unintentional, Juanita negated her partner's effort by redoing the task herself. She didn't accept his work; she rejected/returned it. What's another word for discrediting, rejecting, and negating? *Invalidating.* DUN. DUN. DUNNNNNN. John wasn't reinforced by Juanita's *thank you*; he was punished with invalidation. Similarly, discussing a sexual encounter in couples therapy might not seem problematic, especially if the couple is working on sexual intimacy. But focusing on how someone failed to meet expectations is likely to be experienced as punishing, especially if the individual's "failure" felt like progress to them. Rather than being motivated to try again, the punished partner in this scenario will grow increasingly convinced that the situation is hopeless.

The key to avoiding punishment and fostering change in your partner is to think in terms of small hops or steps and validation. Yes, a grown-ass man should be capable of showing up on time, but your grown-ass man isn't. Accept where you are. Showing up less late than usual is progress. Reinforce it. Or at the very least, don't punish the improvement. Here's where validation becomes invaluable. You might not be able to say that you're glad your partner was still a few minutes late, but you can authentically validate their increased effort and intention to be on time. The beauty of validation is that it forces you to focus on the valid, no matter how imperfect it might be.

Because this is all easier said than done, I'm including examples of validating responses that could have been used to reinforce, or at least not punish, the partners in my previous scenarios:

The Laundry

"Hey, I saw you collected and started all the laundry [Copying]. *Thank you. I see that you are trying to support me and taking what I said to heart* [Proposing]. *You've never been 'all talk' in*

working on us. [Proposing]. *I don't say it enough, but I admire that about you* [Emoting]."

The Sexless Bath

"*I loved the spontaneity of our bath on Tuesday, but I wanted to check in to see if it was overwhelming for you* [Proposing]. *That was a first for us, so it would be totally understandable if it felt awkward* [Equalizing + Proposing]. *We're in this together, babe* [Emoting—implying commitment, loyalty], *and I want to do whatever I can to make this feel good for both of us, even if that means going slowly* [Taking Action]."

The School Supplies

"*I know waiting in long lines in between fighting off angry mobs of back-to-school shoppers isn't a great way to spend time with the kids* [Proposing + Equalizing], *but I see you trying to find ways to support me without my having to ask* [Proposing]. *Thank you, babe.*"

These examples highlight an important point: you don't need to draw attention to any mistakes your partner made to help them do better next time. Are you back? I assume you threw your book because that's typically the type of response I get when I tell people it's okay to reinforce grown adults for doing something partially correct without giving them feedback on what they did wrong. It's true, though: when it comes to making progress, repetition and natural contingencies (e.g., not having dry clothes) are more likely to lead to improvement than criticism or invalidation. The latter simply decreases the chance that your partner will approach the task in the future. Critiques punish attempts; validation reinforces them.

You might also have noticed that in my examples of how to reinforce progress, the reinforcing partner did not express negative emotions. Does that mean you should never express frustration or disappointment? No, of course not. Communicating hurt feelings is fine as long as you don't do it while trying to reinforce change. If, for example, Marcia's priority was to have her partner understand that she was disappointed they didn't have sex, then talking about her hurt would have been the right move. However, when I asked Marcia which was more important, reinforcing progress or having Clara validate her disappointment, she literally laughed out loud. "Obviously, progress! She's all too aware of how disappointed I am with our sex life." It's perfectly reasonable to want people to validate your disappointment and continue to make progress toward meeting your expectations. But because you usually can't do both at the same time, it's up to you to determine which takes priority in any given situation. For what it's worth, focusing your attention on how someone is showing up for you rather than letting you down is likely to decrease your negativity toward them.

Shaping is a process. You're not signing yourself up for a lifetime of moldy clothes by validating your partner's effort and keeping your spot-on critiques to yourself. Once they are consistently helping out more around the house, then you can increase expectations if need be. But I encourage you to think twice before doing so. If you're serious about making changes in your relationship, you will have to accept imperfection. Clothes will be left wet, things will take time, and sales will be missed, but how much does all that matter when you stop and think about it? If you had to choose between efficiency or your relationship, perfection or partnership, acceptance or resentment, which would you choose?

CONFLICT MANAGEMENT

The biggest entry point for punishment in intimate relationships is conflict. Not surprisingly, validating your partner during arguments is among the best things you can do for your relationship. Research suggests that couples who validate each other during conflict are less likely to ice each other out (stonewall) and are more satisfied in their relationships.[2] Communication is better—there's less nagging and fewer instances of saying things that should never ever be said out loud—and fewer problems in the relationship overall. Don't worry if you can't access the higher **Empathy Skills**, like Emoting the sadness you feel on their behalf or Taking Action by compromising your position. According to John Gottman, the nonverbals and basic *Mm-hmms* used in Attending are sufficient.[3]

The dramatic effect validation during conflict has on relationships makes sense if you consider the "5:1 ratio." Research shows that a 5:1 ratio of positivity to negativity during conflict predicts long-term marriage stability, while a ratio of 0.8:1 or lower predicts divorce.[4] Positivity in these studies primarily consisted of validation, even if only through Attending. Negativity was defined as criticism (attacking their character), defensiveness (playing the innocent victim), contempt (disrespecting or degrading them), and stonewalling (refusing to acknowledge or communicate). Gottman coined these behaviors the "Four Horsemen of the Apocalypse" because they correlate with relationship destruction and divorce.[5] I think of them as the four "skills" in an evil doppelgänger's Invalidation Ladder.

Validation is critical to achieving that 5:1 ratio, but in case you haven't tried it, validating someone you're fighting with is So. Freaking. Hard. One comforting fact is that the argument doesn't have to be all sunshine and rainbows. Fights can be heated and messy without being destructive. They can even include invalidation, as long as the ratio of positivity to negativity hovers around 5:1. Remember, simply Attending counts as positivity, and negativity is specific to the Four Horsemen, not expressing negative emotions.

As for how to increase the validation in your arguments, I have two pieces of advice. The first is to finally tattoo "validation ≠ agreement" on your forearm. The tattoo itself won't have any magical properties, but seeing the reminder each day should help you internalize the message.

If you're fighting with someone, it's because you disagree with something they said or did. You're all, "How could you possibly let our six-year-old play *Call of Duty*?!" Disagreement is fine, but if you want to convince the other person of your perspective, or at the very least keep the conversation from becoming stabby, you must find something to validate (e.g., "You love that game almost as much as I love my stand-up comedy podcast, so it makes sense that you'd want to share it with her"). Validation is how you disagree with your partner without disrespecting them.

My other tip on channeling validation during conflicts is to give your partner the benefit of the hurt. The more upset someone becomes, the more hurt you can presume they are. You don't need to agree with the other person's narrative to see that their response to it is real.

Early in my career, I worked with a couple, Sergey and Melinda, both of whom were lawyers. They came to session one day in the midst of an argument about whether or not Sergey had slammed a door on Melinda in frustration. My attempts to direct them toward validation were consistently thwarted by their proclivity for arguing. By the end of the session, they'd each presented airtight cases to prove that Sergey had (or hadn't, from his perspective) slammed the door, but they were angrier than when they arrived.

Years later, I found myself in a similar disagreement with someone over a slammed door, but because he was a cat with no leg to stand on, I couldn't argue with him. Sparrow got spooked when I closed the door after entering his bathroom. From my perspective, I didn't shut the door any louder or more aggressively than I had in the past, but he clearly thought otherwise. He hid and hissed at me, which, of course, meant he was scared. I immediately softened my voice and moved more gently. Because I couldn't reason with him, I had no choice but to accept his reaction.

The other advantage I had when it came to giving Sparrow the benefit of the hurt was that I could see the vulnerability behind his anger and aggression. Anger is often a secondary emotion, meaning it's a reaction to another—aka primary—emotion. With anger, the primary emotion is often fear. A lot of my work with couples comes down to helping them see the fear through the anger they're directing at each other. Beneath Melinda's anger over Sergey slamming the door was her fear that he was losing respect for her. Beneath Sergey's anger over Melinda's accusation was the fear that she would accuse him of violence during an argument. To help you see the small animal that is your partner beneath the puffed-up fur of their anger, ask yourself, "What are they afraid of?" or "How are they feeling threatened?" When anger gets the better of you, asking yourself these questions can help you accurately express your hurt without alienating your partner.

TAKE-HOME POINTS

Punishments are like termites that invisibly eat away at the stability of your relationship. There are several issues that can lead to an infestation of punishment in your intimate partnerships: (1) negative sentiment override, (2) having unrealistic expectations for change, (3) underestimating what might feel punishing, and (4) conflict. The key to avoiding these pitfalls while fostering change is to think in terms of shaping and validation. When your partner fails to meet expectations, look for indications of progress that you could reinforce with validation, and avoid responding in ways that dismiss or minimize their effort. Conflicts are innately punishing, but if you can keep the ratio of validation to invalidation at around 5:1, you'll avoid doing permanent damage to your relationship. To help you maintain this ratio, refer to your validation ≠ agreement tattoo and work on giving your partner the benefit of the hurt.

CHAPTER 17

VALIDATE LIKE A BOSS—
VALIDATION AT WORK

The art of acceptance is the art of making someone who has just done you a
small favor wish that he might have done you a greater one.

—RUSSELL LYNES, *READER'S DIGEST*

When manager Matt Sakaguchi switched to a new team at Google, he wanted to get ahead of the interpersonal problems that plagued his former group.[1] So he did what any self-respecting, overachieving Googler would do—he consulted with researchers on how to establish a healthy team culture. The researchers he spoke with were part of Project Aristotle, an internal division of Google tasked with identifying the key features of high-performing teams. Having studied hundreds of teams and accrued so much data you could probably jump into a pool of it, Scrooge McDuck–style, the researchers at Project Aristotle had some tips for Sakaguchi. They told him he first needed to evaluate his team's strengths and weaknesses. The researchers equipped him with a questionnaire, which he promptly administered to what I can only imagine was a bunch of annoyed employees, because no one wants to fill out *another* questionnaire.

Sakaguchi thought his team was strong, but the survey results suggested otherwise. Faced with disconcerting data, Sakaguchi did what any self-respecting, overachieving manager would do—he arranged for an all-day gathering off-site so his team could discuss the results. He opened the gathering with a clever icebreaker, in which he asked everyone to draw their life's journey, using only pictures to convey how they got to where they are. Sakaguchi went first, and rather than giving the rose-colored glasses timeline you'd expect in a professional setting, he shared (pictorially) that he was suffering from stage IV cancer. Sakaguchi then explained that he'd been undergoing treatment for the last five years while working at Google but that doctors recently discovered a troubling spot on his liver, which meant the cancer might be spreading again. Everyone in the group went on to share their own stories. Rather than crude attempts at re-creating their polished Instagram feeds, participants followed Sakaguchi's lead by depicting their *real* lives, the good and the bad.

Sakaguchi didn't validate an individual with his Disclosure; he validated the universal experience of having a life outside of work. The team's facade of functioning interfered with Sakaguchi's ability to understand the nature of the problems they were facing. He suspected the same thing might be happening on an individual level; he was right. By encouraging people to speak freely, he helped the team see one another, and their problems, more clearly.

Sakaguchi later said, "My goal with that exercise was [for the team] to see that once you hear what people have gone through, you can never look at them the same. You start seeing them as people first, not a co-worker who is making your job harder. At this new level of sharing, we were actually able to get some discussions going about how we can work better as a team. After about a month, the dynamics of the team had changed and it became one of the best teams I've ever worked with at Google."[2]

Sakaguchi wasn't taking his cues from Project Aristotle, at least not directly. None of the researchers with whom he consulted said he should tell the group about his cancer diagnosis, but they did speak to the importance of "psychological safety"—the shared belief by individuals on a team that they won't be invalidated or experience other repercussions (punishments) for asking questions, admitting mistakes, or taking interpersonal risks. In her book *The Fearless Organization*, organizational behaviorist Amy Edmondson broadly defines psychological safety as a "climate in which people are comfortable expressing and being themselves."[3] Having psychological safety within a team means members trust that they can bring their whole selves to work and be accepted.

Researchers at Project Aristotle identified several characteristics of high-performing teams, but psychological safety was far and away the most important.[4] Their research shows that folks on teams high in psychological safety are more likely to stay at the company, earn higher revenue, incorporate diverse ideas from others, and be rated as effective by executives. The importance of psychological safety isn't specific to Google, and the Project Aristotle team wasn't the first to discover it. The concept has been around for decades, and studies in industries ranging from health care to manufacturing have shown that it correlates with innovation, worker engagement, better employee mental health, higher-performing teams, and less turnover.[5]

Sakaguchi's overall approach to establishing psychological safety reads like a page from this book: he *modeled* the behavior he wanted (speaking honestly), provided an opportunity for others to do the same, and then *reinforced* them with validation when they did. Okay, to be fair, I don't know for a fact that Sakaguchi successfully reinforced people with validation. However, considering that his goal was to help folks feel seen and that the team dynamics improved following the off-site, I'm gonna assume some validation went down. At the very least, I'm confident that the majority of the team didn't feel invalidated or *punished* for opening up.

I won't go so far as to say that teams need to be as open as Sakaguchi's to thrive. But I will maintain that establishing psychological safety comes down to validation and a supporting cast of familiar characters—namely, modeling and reinforcement. When validation is modeled and used to reinforce people for taking interpersonal risks, psychological safety increases.

WHEN VALIDATION IS MODELED AND USED TO REINFORCE PEOPLE FOR TAKING INTERPERSONAL RISKS, PSYCHOLOGICAL SAFETY INCREASES.

HOW EMOTIONAL VALIDATION CAN REINFORCE WORKPLACE BEHAVIOR

Validation is the cheapest, sweetest, and most flexible reinforcement you can use in professional settings. It resonates with everyone—trainees, execs, colleagues, customers, managers, etc.—and can reinforce them for anything, from proposing new ideas to returning your stapler. But research suggests that validation in the workplace is seriously lacking. According to a 2017 Gallup poll, only three in ten employees strongly agree with the statement that their opinion matters at work.[6] A separate poll conducted by Catalyst three years later found that nearly half of the women surveyed said they faced difficulties speaking up in virtual meetings, with one in five saying they were overlooked or ignored.[7]

The lack of validation in work settings is an oversight, but it's understandable. Employees are paid to perform for a company. And the expectation is that they'll be routinely evaluated on their ability to do so. When it comes to reinforcement, this culture of evaluation lends itself more to praise than validation. Praise signals positive evaluation or approval (e.g., "Good job," "Nice work," "Great presentation"). The emphasis on being professional—as opposed to personal—means praise is more likely to be focused on the *work* than the person.

There's nothing inherently wrong with praise. I mean, if a person's only mission in life is to gobble it up like the snack pellets in a *PAC-MAN* game, they'll run into some problems, but giving and receiving praise is generally healthy and helpful. Praise is a powerful reinforcement and can easily be used in combination with validation. **"Praise the work; validate the person"** is advice I hear myself giving on an almost weekly basis to my corporate clients. The problem with praise is that when used excessively or not balanced (at least occasionally) with validation, it can seem hollow and impersonal. Impersonal might be what people expect from their interactions at work, but it's not what motivates them.

A study of more than fifteen hundred employees showed that people are *more than three times more likely to be engaged in their work* when they believe their manager cares about their personal life.* [8] Yet less than a third feel their managers actually do. In another survey of more than nine thousand employees across twelve countries, 94 percent agreed with the statement that empathy is "an essential quality for a healthy workplace." Although employees value it, less than half of companies globally provide empathy training. Incidentally, those that do have significantly higher levels of employee engagement.[9]

Your managers, employees, and coworkers value praise; it's just not the only type of communication motivating them. If we've learned anything from clinical research in the last thirty years, it's that validation is conducive to change. It not only helps create a culture that supports creativity and engagement, but also can reinforce specific behaviors. In work settings, validation is particularly well suited to reinforce people for the following:

- Exceeding expectations or making progress in the desired direction.

- Showing tenacity or sustaining progress when other reinforcements are lacking (in the final stretch of a project, following multiple setbacks, etc.).

- Engaging in behaviors that contribute to *psychological safety*, like admitting mistakes, asking for help, and providing feedback.

---

* According to a 2022 Gallup poll, businesses with engaged workers have 23 percent higher profits compared to those with non-engaged workers, as well as significantly lower absenteeism, turnover, and accidents and higher customer loyalty. (Gallup, *State of the Global Workplace Report* [Gallup, 2022], accessed March 1, 2023, https://www .gallup.com/workplace/349484/state-of-the-global-workplace2022-report.aspx.)

For a better sense of how one might use validation to reinforce someone in each of these scenarios, let's look at three real-life examples, only one of which uses real names.

1. Reinforcing a colleague for exceeding expectations and making progress.

My client Pam was the last to say "Not me" when her team was deciding who should speak with their colleague Dwight about his attitude problem. According to Pam, Dwight was "an overbearing hothead," which is why someone needed to give him feedback and why nobody wanted to do it. Dwight had been condescending and dismissive of Pam in the past. She went into the conversation prepared for him to deny responsibility, blame others, and maybe insult her. She did not expect him to be non-defensive and nod along thoughtfully, which is what happened. Pam ended the discussion with praise: "This was a good meeting." We agreed she could have done more to reinforce Dwight's *non-defensiveness* and *receptivity* directly, so she followed up with a short email that I've re-created here:

> *Dwight, I was struck by how non-defensive and receptive you were during our conversation. I don't know if I could have responded with the same level of grace and thoughtfulness to someone giving me difficult feedback* [Equalizing + Caroline Qualifier]. *It was inspiring to see* [Emoting].

2. Reinforcing an employee for showing tenacity and sustaining progress when other reinforcements are lacking.

I hit a lull in my writing earlier this year and sent my editor—also named Caroline—a long email about structural changes I was thinking of making to this book's manuscript. At the end of the email, I said:

I'm afraid this book sucks. Like, really sucks. Please tell me if it does. I won't be offended. I'm good at self-validation, so even if my feelings get hurt, I can validate them and feel better. 😅

Caroline's response:

First, I have read a large part of this manuscript, and it most definitely did not suck. So unless you've rewritten the whole thing, it is impossible for it to 100 percent suck [praise].
  Second, being convinced at this point that it sucks is TOTALLY NORMAL. This happens to all writers at about this stage. I might be more concerned at this point if you didn't think it sucked. It's like literary puberty—unpleasant but unavoidable [validation—Equalizing].

This email is a solid example of praising the work while validating the person. Caroline's response shook me out of my lull, enabling me to pick up my writing pace again. She also reinforced me for taking interpersonal risks—asking for honest feedback, expressing emotions, and using humor. Her words made me more inclined to bring "my whole self" to our conversations moving forward.*

3. Reinforcing a colleague for behaviors that build psychological safety.

Michael, a director I was collaborating with on a mental health initiative, made some comments that felt, shall we say, privileged. I decided to email him to say I was offended and express my concerns. Alienating the director would have been a disaster for the

---

* In case you're wondering, no, I did not reinforce Caroline for praising and validating me by praising and validating her in return. We already have the same name, and her ability to use validation as reinforcement (although effective) freaked me out a little. There's a decent chance Caroline is me from the future.

initiative, but it was a risk I was willing to take. He responded immediately:

> *I hate when I'm worried I've offended someone in an email and am then stuck waiting all day for them to respond, so I wanted to get back to you asap, even though I can only fire off a few points* [Equalizing and Taking Action].
>
> 1. *You did NOT offend me with your feedback; you informed me.*
> 2. *I now see how insensitive my comments were* [Equalizing—he's suggesting anyone in my shoes would feel the same way].
> 3. *I'm embarrassed by what I said. More importantly, I hate that I hurt you* [Emoting]. *I want to make this right* [Taking Action].
>   *More soon!*

Michael probably realized he needed to respond sensitively to my email, given the nature of the issue I raised, but I don't think he ran his response by HR before pressing send. He was speaking from the heart, like Pam and Caroline in the previous examples. Herein lies an important point: you don't need a detailed list of things you're hoping people will spontaneously do so you can reinforce them with validation; your emotions will cue you into these opportunities. Pam was *shocked* by Dwight's response; Caroline *empathized* with where I was at. If a colleague says or does something that evokes strong positive emotions within you, reinforcement à la validation might be in order. Importantly, strong negative emotions, like what I imagine Michael felt, also can be an indication that you need to reinforce someone with validation. We typically feel attacked when people are trying to hurt us, but we also may feel attacked when they're trying to stop us from hurting them.

The sense of mischaracterization and indignation we experience when we're called out is our ego's knee-jerk reaction to being put in its place. These fighty emotions are secondary to the hurt of having hurt someone and the fear of what that means for our character, relationship, and work. The mind's natural response to all this negativity is to spin up an egocentric, defensive narrative to protect you ("They're so sensitive!" "That's not what I meant!"). Instead, these negative emotions and the thoughts surrounding them should serve as your cue to go looking for kernels of truth. The other person might be operating on misinformation or unrealistic expectations, but focusing on what they got wrong is as easy as it is counterproductive. You may disagree with others' interpretations, but if you want people to tell you if you've offended them, you need to find some way to reinforce them when they do.

I chose to end on Michael's example because it highlights the relationship between the main themes in this chapter—psychological safety, validation as reinforcement, and diversity and inclusion, which we turn to now.

PUTTING THE INCLUSION IN DIVERSITY AND INCLUSION

Acceptance by a group is not simply a matter of being admitted into that group. A business might not show any discrimination in its hiring practices but consistently underpay or tolerate microaggressions toward minorities such that they feel alienated or undervalued. Inclusion requires representation *and* acceptance. True to form, industries in the Western world have been mostly concerned with appearances ("Are we hiring enough women of color?") and not experiences ("Do the women we've hired feel included?"). Far from encouraging acceptance, our approach to diversity has historically been to ignore it. Until recently, "I don't see color"* was considered an enlightened perspective, and most institutions were operating under the mistaken belief that minority groups would joyously assimilate into the majority through some metaphorical

---

* The word *color* can be replaced with *gender, age, disability, neurodiversity,* etc.

melting pot—an image that is as disturbing as the concept it represents.

Over time, it's become increasingly clear that the way to foster inclusion isn't to ignore our differences. It's to acknowledge them, nonjudgmentally; some might say mindfully, with understanding and empathy such that another person feels accepted. On the heels of the Black Lives Matter and #MeToo movements, institutions have become increasingly called upon to recognize experiences they once ignored.

The biggest obstacle they face now is fear. People are avoiding conversations about diversity and inclusion, not because they think it's productive to do so, but for fear that their lack of understanding will make matters worse. As problematic as the fear is, I see a silver lining in the fact that people are thinking long and hard about how to communicate acceptance and safeguard against invalidation. I mean, how many times in history has that been the case? If you were to walk through my local bookstore, you'd think there was a Golden Ticket buried inside books on diversity and inclusion because they are flying off the shelves. The question everyone seems to be trying to answer nowadays is, how do you talk about experiences you can't relate to? **In other words, how can you validate someone if you don't understand or empathize with their experience?**

Reader, because you're well on your way to earning an honorary degree from the Caroline School of Validation, why don't you take a shot at answering this question? Hint: refer to the Validation Ladder's framework. If you said, "Use the **Mindfulness Skills**," congratulations! You've officially earned your degree.

I don't mean to reduce the complexity of dialoguing about diversity and inclusion to a couple of skills. There's a lot to consider in these conversations. The problems and solutions we face are complicated, but in honor of dialectics, I want to balance the complexity with some simplicity: the first step toward communicating acceptance is to develop and demonstrate awareness. The **Mindfulness Skills**, Attending and Copying, can help you do just that. These skills are designed to immerse you in another person's experience. They are not a substitute for education or cultural immersion, but they offer a meaningful first step toward understanding and empathy.

In closing this discussion, I want to appeal to leaders and those of you in positions of power to make a point of using your validation skills at work, because you may be in the strongest position to influence diversity and inclusion. A study of more than twenty thousand students across thirty-four different colleges in the United States found that interpersonal and academic validation from faculty and staff directly affected the degree to which students felt a sense of belonging and—wait for it—that these experiences helped offset the negative effects of discrimination and bias.* [10] In the authors' words, "The validating experiences can reinforce self-worth and value in educational environments that may help students remain resilient despite microaggressions and assaults on their social identity."[11] Meanwhile, research suggests that managers with strong interpersonal skills like validation are seen by their direct reports as being more supportive of diversity and inclusiveness.[12] As one researcher noted, "an ounce of genuine, open-minded acceptance is worth more than a pound of affirmative action policies, politically correct internal communications, and diversity education programs."[13]

The effects reported in these studies are impressive, but they mostly affirm something we already knew: people in positions of power are powerful. This is not to say that the rest of us are powerless, but simply that those in a position to hire or fire, pass or fail, have a responsibility to include and accept, reinforce and validate.

---

* "Academic validation" is defined by the authors as affirming someone's inner capacity to learn and be in college. It includes behaviors like attending to students by encouraging their questions and participation and demonstrating care and concern for their progress.

CHAPTER 18

EVERYBODY HURTS— SELF-VALIDATION

[The] curious paradox is that when I accept myself as I am, then I change.
—CARL ROGERS, *ON BECOMING A PERSON*

It's New Year's Eve night, and I'm alone at home, writing. Mat and Havana are in Washington, visiting my awesome in-laws. I want to be with my family, but I couldn't make the trip. Flying has triggered multiple sclerosis (MS) flares for me in the past. For the record, an MS flare is characterized by the worsening of existing symptoms or the onset of new symptoms. Basically, it's like spilling water on your computer, except the water is some unknown trigger in the environment, and the computer is your brain.

I experienced an unexpected flare last month, so I can't risk another. I thought about driving to Seattle, but the muscle spasms that still haven't resolved from the previous flare make it impossible for me to be seated for very long. I type furiously for thirty minutes and then drop and do my push-up/jumping jacks combo. It would take me two years to drive to Seattle at this pace, not to mention enough bizarre side-of-the-road calisthenics to get me locked away somewhere.

While writing, I notice a darkness inside me. I can feel it swirling in my chest, constricting my throat, and pressing behind my eyes. The lyrics from a Dave Matthews Band song are bouncing around my head, "Why are you different? Why are you that way?"[1]

It feels vulnerable and reckless to share my experience with you. And not just the part about still listening to the Dave Matthews Band. Books like mine are supposed to be relatable, but I've yet to meet another person with my strange cocktail of symptoms and limitations. I've decided to roll with the vulnerability and share my story because the reality is that everyone struggles with negative emotions and the invalidating thoughts that inflate them.

We tend to confuse feeling bad with being bad. But there's nothing wrong or abnormal about having emotions like loneliness and insecurity. Everybody hurts, and everybody experiences the same flavor of hurt at some point or another. Interestingly, the ways we invalidate ourselves also are more or less the same. When we experience setbacks, our negative core beliefs get activated. Negative core beliefs are essentially invalidating self-concepts that we *know* deep down are true. I mean, they're not actually true, but the rigid way we cling to them sure makes it seem like they are. People develop these beliefs in response to painful experiences in childhood, and you should pity the fool (or therapist) who tries to challenge them, because they are often central to a person's identity.[2]

You'd expect people's negative core beliefs to be as diverse as the experiences, cultures, and upbringings that inform them. Au contraire. Research suggests that the invalidating beliefs people maintain about themselves generally fall into one of three categories: helplessness (e.g., "I'm needy"), unlovability (e.g., "I'm defective"), and worthlessness (e.g., "I'm toxic").[3] Our experiences might differ, but the emotions we feel and the ways we invalidate ourselves are common.

Working through the various forms of self-invalidation that compound suffering is what this chapter is about. I don't want to bum you out with my lame health stuff (too late?), but I also don't want to make up a scenario or recall a situation with the swagger of having already processed it. For one thing, I'm clearly a fan of teaching through modeling, and I prioritize authenticity over perfection whenever possible. For another, I'm a big DIYer and hate nothing more than a YouTube video of someone fast-forwarding through the tricky parts of a project to showcase the end result from twelve different angles. I want to see what they do when the IKEA shelves they're using to transform a closet collapse in on them and puncture a floorboard.

The negativity I'm feeling about being alone on New Year's Eve is real, as is the self-invalidation that's amplifying it. In this final chapter, we'll look at the phenomena of self-invalidation and challenge it with—you guessed it—self-validation. I'll explain how to apply the validation skills you've learned in this book to help you direct mindfulness, understanding, and care to difficult emotions like regret and despair, which can seem dangerous to acknowledge, much less accept.

SELF-INVALIDATION

Seeing the error in your ways isn't the same as invalidating yourself. Self-invalidation occurs when you adopt a harsh, self-critical stance toward your mistakes or perceived shortcomings (e.g., "I'm such an idiot") or internalize them as character flaws (e.g., "This makes me unlovable"). Judging, dismissing, trivializing, or doubting your emotions and internal experiences also constitutes self-invalidation. Although invalidating your emotions is meant to deny them, suffering doesn't play by vampire rules. It doesn't need an invitation to come inside, and if you slam the door in its face, it might leave, but only so it can go grab some friends to help it break down the door. Those "friends" include shame, disgust, and self-loathing.

In response to the virtual house party of negativity that results from self-invalidation, we either try to avoid thinking about the situation that led to our emotions or get bizarrely defensive—*with ourselves*—in an attempt to justify whatever we thought, felt, or did. The result is a ruminative cycle that might seem like introspection but couldn't be farther from it. Whereas introspection is intentional and nonjudgmental, rumination is obsessive, uncontrollable, and incriminatory. **Introspection fosters growth; rumination stifles it.**

Self-validation, on the other hand, is an accepting response toward one's suffering and the mistakes, urges, compulsions, addictions, transgressions, and shortcomings that contributed to it. Rather than raising doubts about or minimizing one's own internal experiences, self-validation affirms them. Studies have shown that self-validation and self-compassion, far from leading to a giant pity party, are associated with decreased rumination and neuroticism.[4] Self-validators also report increased motivation to repair and avoid repeating misdeeds, compared to those who do not validate themselves, and are more likely to view their perceived shortcomings as changeable.[5]

To reiterate a point I've made repeatedly in part 3, excessive punishment wreaks havoc on relationships and the well-being of those exposed to it. That includes punishments you levy against yourself. Whatever guilt, sadness, or disappointment you feel is more than enough to help you learn from your mistakes. You don't need to waterboard yourself with negativity to stay on the straight and narrow. Unfortunately, self-invalidation has become like a dominant gene passed down from generation to generation. Most of us suffer from self-invalidation to some degree. It's just a matter of how much and whether we have the skills to manage it.

THE SKILLS

Self-validation is about bringing mindfulness, understanding, and empathy to your emotions and experiences so that you can accept them. The approach I developed uses the basic framework of the Validation Ladder and was informed by Christopher Germer and Kristin Neff's work on self-compassion and Dialectical Behavior Therapy's distress tolerance techniques.[6]

Because you're communicating with yourself, a couple of the skills from the Validation Ladder won't apply. Reading your own mind isn't particularly meaningful, so you can take Proposing off the list. The same goes for Disclosure, presuming you're not moved by hearing things you already know about yourself.

The six remaining skills—Attending, Copying, Contextualizing, Equalizing, Emoting, and Taking Action—are the steps to self-validation, and you'll move through all of them. Rather than using whichever skills feel natural and accessible to you, self-validation has you begin with the **Mindfulness Skills** and progress sequentially through the skills as I've listed them.* Although mindfulness is the starting point, you can return to these skills whenever you get distracted or overwhelmed.

If it feels cheesy or unnatural to direct certain skills to yourself, remember, *that's why you're doing this.* Learning to tolerate and evolve past the discomfort takes time and patience. As with any new skill set, the more you practice, the more you'll take to it.

In the next section, I move between describing what to do and modeling how to do it by applying the skills to myself. I target just one emotion, but in practice, you can focus on more than one. At the end of this chapter, you'll find a self-validation exercise that will walk through each of the six steps I describe.

MINDFULNESS SKILLS—WHAT AM I FEELING?

In self-validation, the **Mindfulness Skills** help you feel your emotions without feeding them.

Step 1: Attending

To Attend, you'll again use nonverbals, listen, and ask questions to cultivate awareness. Rather than signaling that you're paying attention, you want to communicate acceptance right out of the gate.

---

* Close readers might notice that Emoting comes after Taking Action in the Validation Ladder, but is listed before it here. The reason is that the skills in each skill set are interchangeable when it comes to validating others. Each skill set is more challenging and powerful than the preceding one(s), but the skills in each skill set themselves aren't listed in any particular order. When validating others, however, order is important, and Emoting should come before Taking Action.

The Big Four nonverbals* won't help you here, but *opening your palms, relaxing your body,* and *deepening your breath* will. These nonverbal cues counter the fight/flight/freeze response your body assumes when it's trying to protect you. Through the remarkable channels of biofeedback, your nervous system will start to get the message that it can relax and decrease its resistance to the enemy, which in this case is you yourself.

> *I'm currently sitting hunched over and typing with my legs crossed. Time to see if I can send a message to my nervous system that reads: "Chill the F out." In truth, I don't feel much tension or resistance, just the swirling darkness I mentioned earlier. Regardless, I will cross my arms and clench all my muscles for twenty to thirty seconds and then release them. Note: this is a classic trick therapists use to help clients relax muscles they might not have realized they were tensing. After I let go, I'll sit with my palms up and limbs uncrossed while taking ten deep breaths from my diaphragm. Here goes.*
>
> *Okay, I'm back, and it turns out my body was totally lying earlier when it said I wasn't feeling tense. I was holding on to a lot. Also, I hurt my back from clenching too hard. Note to reader: don't clench too hard. Note to self: don't judge yourself for clenching too hard.*

For the listening component of Attending, you'll use a modified version of the A Game to help you get to the heart of what you're experiencing. When it comes to yourself, the "heart" will always be the emotion(s) surrounding whatever problem you're grappling with. **So instead of asking, "Why does this matter?" the question you need to answer is, "What am I feeling?"** Easier said than done. Emotions are like the social media account of a celebrity whose password is 1234. The real emotion will be posting things like, "I'm frustrated," or "I'm annoyed," and then a judgment will hack into

---

* Eye contact, proximity, gesturing, nodding.

the account and post, "I'm an idiot." If you mindlessly scroll through the feed, you'll mistake the judgment for the emotion, but it's an imposter. To Attend to your *emotions*, you must filter out the judgments, negative interpretations, projections, and other thoughts that seem like feelings but are really just reactions to them. **Feelings are called feelings because you can feel them.** Try to locate the emotion in your body, and sit with it. When you've identified an emotion, label it using an emotion adjective to help differentiate it from the hacks.

I close my eyes in search of a feeling to describe the swirling darkness I've been trying to ignore. "I'm broken" is the first thing that comes to mind. That's a judgment. "No, it's not," insists the judgment. "It's a fact. You can't do what other people do. You can't even sit through a movie. Broken." Feel, don't feed, I tell myself. The judgment passes like a cloud. I listen to my body, to the aching swelling in my chest, the dull threat of tears behind my eyes. I feel it in my heart, the sense of falling while sitting still. This is despair.

Step 2: Copying

As soon as you identify an emotion (e.g., despair), your mind will send in swarms of Green Beret–caliber thoughts to obscure it and beat you up. They pull out the big guns—painful memories from childhood, elaborate explanations of why you suck, lyrics from old Dave Matthews Band songs—anything to distract you from the feeling while expertly exacerbating it. **To help sustain mindful awareness under these conditions, Copy or repeat the emotion.** Saying it out loud or writing it down can help increase awareness by engaging more parts of the brain. To protect against overidentifying with the feeling, describe it using "this is" as opposed to "I am" language (e.g., "This is anger," as opposed to "I am angry"). Despite the emphasis on "self," self-validation helps you recognize the humanity in your suffering. The personal narrative that tries to attach itself to your emotions creates the illusion that you are alone in your experience. "Nobody could possibly relate to my strange cocktail of symptoms and limitations." Beneath the illusion that you're different is the reality that you're human.

> *The instant I identify despair, the troops swarm in. I'm attacked with thoughts, "You've got a fully stocked refrigerator and a MacBook; you don't know the first thing about despair." And memories—an email from my brother fifteen years ago in which he called me selfish; California's bright sun sprawled across the bed where I lay, utterly exhausted at eleven a.m., listening to neighbors returning home from the farmers market. "This is despair," I repeat to myself, trying to feel the emotion without feeding it. Easier said than done. Thoughts about the emotion keep distracting me. I Copy the words "This is despair" in the Notes app on my phone. I repeat them to myself. Eventually, the space between my thoughts and feelings expands. The more I focus on feeling the emotion, the duller it becomes.*

UNDERSTANDING: WHY AM I FEELING THIS WAY?

The **Understanding Skills** focus your attention on *facts*, not fault, so you can examine the validity of your emotions without spiraling into shame and blame. Note: I discuss Contextualizing and Equalizing separately, but in practice, you can toggle between them.

Steps 3 and 4: Contextualizing

With Contextualizing, you're again looking for the trail of cause and effect that leads to a reaction. Here, the reaction you're solving for is your emotion and the *facts* to consider are the circumstances that may have prompted or exacerbated it, including past events, misinformation, and disorder. The "past" includes events in the recent past like having received a disparaging email from a colleague and vulnerability factors like having skipped lunch or not having slept well.

Assumptions and judgments are often misleading, so you can consider them misinformation for this exercise. Don't chastise yourself for making assumptions or having judgments; simply recognize them for what they are and how they affect you. **Contextualizing acknowledges the conditions that contribute to your emotions without blaming yourself or others for them.**

I enjoy being alone; I prefer the sound of keys typing to people talking, so why am I feeling despair? "I have MS" seems too obvious, so I look back at what I've written so far for hints. Interesting. The thoughts and memories I've recorded suggest other causes for my despair—I'm selfish, ungrateful, and perhaps overdramatic. ~~Don't let yourself off the hook for this stuff!~~ These thoughts aren't facts. What are the facts?

- *I am not choosing to be at home. The fact of the matter is that traveling could jeopardize my health. Also, I'm in pain. Pain often leads to despair. #disorder*
- *My symptoms have prevented me from doing many things I wanted to do during the years. The disappointment doesn't go away just because the moment has passed. #history*
- *I've been judging myself harshly for struggling with this disorder. I appear to assume that because there's something wrong, there must be something wrong with me. #misinformation*

Turns out the obvious answer—I have MS—was the correct one. For the millionth time, I'm reminded that acceptance isn't an achievement you can cross off a list; it's a practice. "My name is Caroline Fleck, and I have MS."

Steps 3 and 4: Equalizing

In the earlier chapter on Equalizing, I encouraged you to use the Golden Rule approach of putting yourself in another person's shoes to help you understand and validate them. Equalizing your own experiences requires the opposite: you must recognize the humanity in your emotions. We presume that certain negative feelings—jealousy, anger, despair, etc.—reflect poorly on our character and are unacceptable. But these are normal emotions that all people experience. It might be problematic to act on them, but you don't need to beat yourself up with invalidation when they arise. To Equalize your emotions, look at the facts beneath the perfectionistic standards and expectations you've internalized. **Ask yourself, would I judge a friend for feeling what I'm feeling in this situation? How would I respond to a loved one if they were in my shoes?**

*I ask myself if I'd negatively judge my brother-in-law, Joe, who has Crohn's disease, for feeling despair if his symptoms prevented him from traveling. The answer is a visceral "NO!" The judgment is so discordant with how I'd respond to him that it feels offensive and gross. Okay, so if it would be understandable for Joe to feel despair, why not me? "Because you're a psychologist." What. The. Hell. Mind, please explain yourself. "I don't know, shouldn't you have graduated from emotions like despair?" No. Psychologists, like all people, are allowed to feel despair. Would I judge any of my colleagues for experiencing despair? Another visceral "NO!" So? "So, you're different from and weaker than they are." I'm going to return to the **Mindfulness Skills** for a bit. "Yeah, I figured that was coming." I'm back. So, the facts are these:*

- *I wouldn't judge my family or colleagues for feeling despair.*
- *All people feel despair, even psychologists.*
- *If another person were in my shoes, I'd have empathy for them.*

At this point, I can see where the despair is coming from, and I'm about 95 percent convinced that it's a reasonable reaction to the circumstances.

EMPATHY SKILLS: HOW CAN I SHOW CARE AND COMPASSION TOWARD MYSELF?

The **Empathy Skills** help you respond to your suffering with kindness and channel it toward something constructive. If it's confusing to think about applying empathy to yourself, you can replace the term with *compassion,* or *compassionate empathy* as it's sometimes called. According to Paul Ekman, compassion is a subset of empathy that is specific to suffering and reflected in the urge to reduce it.[7]

Step 5: Emoting

When Emoting to validate others, you express your feelings in response to what someone has shared. **In self-validation, the emotions you express toward yourself are** *care* **and** *compassion.* Once again, you will rely on verbal and nonverbal communication to Emote. Note: don't be fooled into thinking you can skip Emoting because you're too cool for self-talk. You've been talking to yourself for decades, just not very nicely.

Touch—be it through hugs, held hands, or patted backs—is among the most common nonverbal ways we demonstrate care for others. In self-validation, you'll use similar gestures to comfort yourself. Everyone's relationship with their body is different, so experiment with various gestures to find one that feels comforting and supportive to you. Examples include the following:

- Hugging yourself while stroking your arms
- Placing one hand over your heart
- Patting or resting one hand on your stomach
- Cradling one hand in the other

When speaking to yourself, focus on phrases that are simple and kind. Avoid self-affirmations like, "I'm good enough, I'm smart enough, and gosh darn it, people like me." The intention is to express tenderness toward your emotions without trying to change them.* Examples include the following:

- This is hard.
- I forgive you.
- May I accept what I cannot change.
- I love you.

As soon as I place my right hand on my stomach, I feel an immediate sense of ease and openness—perhaps a classically conditioned response after all these years of pairing the gesture with kindness. I imagine myself crouched down and patting the back of a woman who matches my description. I know the woman is me, but not seeing her face provides enough of a disconnect for me to experience the empathy I'd naturally feel toward someone in despair. "Let it be," I tell her. Sometimes I say, "I love you," to comfort myself, but those words don't come naturally right now. As I sit here on New Year's Eve, the words are, "Let it be." "Let it be, hon," I repeat with warmth and assuredness. "Just let it be."

Step 6: Taking Action

If you take your emotions seriously, it stands to reason that you should respond seriously to them, too; self-soothing and making meaning are two ways to do so. The gateway to self-soothing is through the senses—taste, touch, smell, sight, and sound. Examples include drinking warm tea, taking a bath, lighting candles, tidying your space, and listening to relaxing music. These activities are intended to make your suffering easier to bear, not deny or amplify it.

---

* Responding with tenderness toward your emotions without trying to change them will end up changing your emotions for the better. But if you're only trying to feel better, you'll see through yourself because you are yourself, and it won't work. I realize we've transcended into Yoda logic, but trust me, it all checks out.

If I was trying to care for someone in despair, I'd eventually help
them off of the floor and make them some tea. So that's exactly
what I'm going to do. I'll also light my trusty Paddywax
Yosemite-scented candle, grab the soft Squishmallow I
sometimes use as a pillow, play some Chopin, and start a fire.

Okay, I'm back. I'm feeling less raw now, despite running
into some issues, like spilling hot tea on my hands and
getting into an all-out shouting match with Google Home,
which took my voice command to play Chopin as an excuse to
blast "Chopsticks" at top volume. Despite the obstacles, I feel
better, calmer.

Making meaning from negative emotions and experiences is possible only once you've decreased the self-invalidation that punishes you out of accepting them. I've always looked at suffering as energy. It can be used for constructive or destructive purposes, but the energy itself is neutral. If you don't accept the painful things you've done or that have been done to you, then you don't get a say in how that energy gets directed. Left to its own devices, negativity often ends up fueling self-destructive behavior. We're so afraid of wallowing in our emotions that we end up wallowing in our attempts to avoid them.

Accepting suffering doesn't mean it will subsume or define you; through acceptance, you can define it. **Taking Action has you channel the tender emotions you've been holding in ways that bring meaning to your life.** Pick up a neglected instrument, read an article on an issue you care about, bake someone cookies, or pour your heart out into writing a chapter about self-validation in the hope that another person reads and finds it helpful. It doesn't matter how big or small; just take a step toward something that matters to you, and let it be a step you did not plan to take that day.

The chapter is one thing, but my heart is telling me I need to
email a woman I met at Petco back in July. She runs a nonprofit

that places foster animals in local pet stores to help get them
adopted, and I've been meaning to reach out to see if she needs
any help with the daily caretaking. Yes, I realize it's been more
than six months; no, I don't know why it's taken me so long to
contact her. All I know is I don't want to write an email right
now. I'm exhausted and in pain. Blah, blah, blah. Okay,
let's do this.

And I'm back. I offered to help out on Thursday and
Sunday evenings with Havana. I have to say, I feel good.
Really good, actually. Writing the email didn't exhaust or tax
me like I thought it would. It reminded me of my strength.
I cannot fly to Seattle right now, but I can still empty
a litter box.

SELF-VALIDATION EXERCISE

Practice this exercise during periods of distress or vulnerability. I
highly recommend writing out your responses to the questions until you've memorized the process and can go through each step
without getting distracted.

If you get distracted at any point in this practice, use the **Mindfulness Skills** to ground you.

FAMOUS LAST WORDS

Like all writers, I relied on the literary equivalent of a glam squad
to help me polish my chapters after I wrote them. My squad of
readers and editors was responsive, thoughtful, and generally patient with the many editorial mistakes I made along the way, but
there was one issue I think everyone grew sick of flagging: inconsistent pronouns. To clarify, I wasn't confusing gender pronouns,
which can seriously invalidate a person's identity and should be
avoided at all costs. No, my problem was of the "I"/"you" variety. I
used "they" and "we" interchangeably, and the "I" referenced at
the beginning of a sentence was often a "you" by the end. For

Mindfulness: What Am I Feeling?	**Step 1: Attend**	· Squeeze all your muscles and then open your palms, relax your body, and deepen your breath. · Ask yourself, "What am I feeling?" Focus on where you experience the emotion in your body, and label your feelings using emotion adjectives (frustrated, scared, sad, etc.).
	Step 2: Copy	· Pull your attention away from any thoughts that arise, and return your focus to your feelings. · Repeat "This is [emotion you identified]" to yourself like a mantra, or write down the phrase.
Understanding: Why Am I Feeling This Way?	**Steps 3 and 4: Contextualizing and Equalizing**	**Contextualizing:** Consider the larger context in which your emotions are occurring—the past (recent and distant), misinformation (including assumptions and judgments), disorder, etc. **Equalizing:** Ask yourself: · Would I judge a friend for feeling what I'm feeling in this situation? · How would I respond to a close friend if they were in my shoes?

Empathy: How Can I Show Care and Compassion Toward Myself?	**Step 5: Emote**	· Experiment with various forms of gentle touch. Examples include the following:
		  - Placing one hand over your heart
		  - Hugging yourself while stroking your arms
		  - Touching or gently rubbing your stomach
		  - Cradling one hand in the other
		· Speak kind words to yourself as though you were comforting a friend. Use simple and comforting phrases like, "I love you," or "This is hard."

	Step 6: Take Action	· Self-soothe by attending to your five senses. · Do something that reflects your values, such as attending to others, creating art, exercising, or reading. Note: choose something you weren't already planning to do.

example, I wrote: "Yes, I aim to validate someone, not get a ticker-tape parade for my efforts, but if the person treats you worse over time, or you don't feel good about yourself after intervening, back way off of this skill."

Over time, the "inconsistent pronouns" comment was reduced to "pronouns," and eventually "pronouns!!!!!" as the issue persisted. Too bad, so sad for my glam squad, because no amount of feedback kept me from repeating these mistakes over and over again.

The tendency to swap I/you pronouns is a bad habit I seem to have developed over the years. Or is it? I'm not one to psychoanalyze slips of the tongue (or keyboard), but part of me likes to believe that I was subconsciously confusing pronouns on purpose to make a point: namely, that we're one and the same. It's a cheesy point, but one that I grow more convinced of each day.

My work on validation has led me to focus less on the characteristics that divide people—husband versus wife, boss versus employee, psychologist versus feral cat—and more on the connections between them. Where once I saw an infinite chasm separating "you" from "me," now I see a small valley with bridges running across it. My hurt hurts you. Validating others serves us, and validating ourselves serves others. Maybe my pronoun swaps were a subconscious attempt to underscore these points. Maybe I'm just a sloppy writer. Or maybe they were an act of defiance.

When pitching my book proposal to agents and publishers, some expressed concerns about the book's emphasis on others. Or rather, the emphasis on *accepting* others. No one took issue with a book about changing others. Those books sell like McDonald's breakfast sandwiches. The question was if readers would be up for focusing first and foremost on acceptance. In the terrain of self-help, would a book about validating others stand a chance? I believed it could. Especially because the whole premise is that acceptance leads to change. Not to mention the fact that accepting others is a form of self-help. Solitary confinement and social isolation are considered torture because connection with others is critical to our growth and stability. It just so happens that, next to solitary confinement, failing to accept people is the surest way to become alienated from them.

Still, I get it. Acceptance isn't as sexy as change, even if it amounts to change in the end. Actually, I don't get it. That's just what I was told. I believe acceptance and change are two sides of the same coin. I believe that working on how we relate to others is often the easiest way to change how we relate to ourselves and that it's in our best interest to confuse "you" with "me" from time to time, albeit not when writing a book. Lastly, I believe in people like you, who see that validating others serves you and validating yourself serves others.

Thanks to the tireless and much-needed help of my glam squad, the pronoun slips have all been corrected (I think). But I didn't want the points they may have reflected to be lost. To do justice to the ideas that informed my work on validation, I'll leave you with the words of those who capture the spirit of my perspective and inspire me to this day.

The more one forgets himself—by giving himself to
a cause to serve or another person to love—the more human
he is and the more he actualizes himself.

—VIKTOR FRANKL[8]

You and me
are us and them, and it and sky.

—ADA LIMÓN[9]

Acceptance is the first step toward change.

—MARSHA LINEHAN[10]

EPILOGUE

I have no boobs. I mean, I do, but they're not mine. Mine were taken during a double mastectomy in the summer of 2023. What I have now are metal expanders filled with saline. And breast cancer. I was diagnosed exactly one week after putting the final period on the final sentence on what should have been the final page of this book.

Editing my manuscript during chemotherapy has been surreal. Statements like, "I never wanted to give a disease anything it hadn't already taken from me," seem more foreboding than inspirational now that my hair is falling out in clumps. And I'm struck by how much distance I had from the difficult experiences I was describing. Yes, the MS symptoms are active, but the diagnosis itself is old news. Yes, the flares are all different, but I understand what they are and have established workarounds to help me manage them so that most people are none the wiser. Like a werewolf, I've been able to maintain appearances while periodically slipping into the shadows to ride out various symptoms and treatments. This combination of self-reliance and compartmentalization has allowed me to focus on my two full-time jobs: mom and psychologist. For most of my adult life, I've been more of a caretaker than a care-receiver.

Cancer changed all that. Unlike depression and MS, which I was fortunate enough to be able to manage independently and hide as needed, cancer can't be concealed with a breezy smile and a makeshift fort under my desk where I can crash between clients. For the first time in my life, I look as bad as I feel. There's no way to camouflage the tubes draining fluid from my chest wall as I walk to the farmers market or the translucent-green hue of my skin from chemotherapy. People aren't saying, "But you seem so healthy" like they did when I told them I have MS. Instead, everyone's eyes get all round and anime when they talk to me, like they're looking at a forsaken animal at the pound.

Fortunately, being on the receiving end of so much attention and care hasn't changed any of the perspectives I champion in this book. If anything, cancer has reinforced my belief that making meaning out of suffering by using it to connect with and validate others brings us as close as we can ever be to what some call "enlightenment." However, reading back over the manuscript with the hindsight of these last few months, I realize there are two points that did not get sufficient airtime. The first is that self-validation is like a Captain America–caliber shield against external invalidation.

From clients to doctors, to the neighbor whose aunt was recently diagnosed with stage III, everyone who knows I have cancer—which, again, is everyone—seems to be an expert on what to expect and how to prepare. "The first week after chemo is the hardest." "My cousin said you need a handheld showerhead for after the mastectomy." "Take the pain meds they give you." Sometimes their expectations are communicated as directives. My oncologist told me to take a minimum of four months off of work for chemo as though paid medical leave was a given for someone being treated at Stanford. The surgeon said I shouldn't elevate my heart rate for eight weeks following the mastectomy. When it was my turn to order at an ice cream parlor, a family member quickly announced, "She'll just have water," before whispering, "Sugar feeds cancer," to me in a tone I've heard used only in movies when one character tells the other to "Act natural."

For the most part, I generally appreciate people's recommendations and insights (except when they stand between me and ice cream). The problem is that everyone is so convinced about what's right that discerning what's right *for me* would be near impossible if I didn't already have a self-validation practice. At night or, let's be honest, midday as I lie cocooned under my comforter, I mentally climb the steps of my Self-Validation Ladder to ascertain what I'm feeling, why I'm feeling it, and what I need moving forward. Sometimes I rely on the wisdom I've gleaned from others; sometimes I do the exact opposite of what they suggest. Either way, I feel confident in my decisions.

Self-validation also has the handy-dandy feature of being able to shield you from the sense of invalidation that naturally arises when the world seems to be insisting that your feelings are "wrong." For instance, in the seventy-two hours after my chemotherapy treatments, I experience depersonalization, wherein it seems like I'm observing myself from outside my body. Mat can attest to the fact that, despite being a psychologist, I suck at describing what this feels like. The best I've got is that it's a combination of angsty agitation and distress resulting from the sense that I am not myself. Cats are not cute. Stand-up is annoying. It's a real drag. I'm not depressed or apathetic so much as absent. The only hint of "me" is the awareness that I am not as I have always been.

An unexpected disdain for kittens is not listed anywhere in the pages and pages of printouts my oncologist gave me on the side effects of chemotherapy. The doctors and nurses I've talked to about this depersonalization have all responded with some version of "I've never heard of that," before quickly moving on to something else. Translation: "That's not valid."

In the absence of self-validation, I would have doubted myself. "Maybe it's not the chemo? Maybe there's something wrong with me?" Being able to see the validity in my emotions and trusting in my experience over others' expectations has protected me from what I can only imagine would have been a smorgasbord of self-invalidation. There are times in my life when I would have thought I was crazy or overdramatic or even questioned my experience. Basically, there are times in my life when I would have reacted toward myself as society often reacts to women's medical symptoms—by dismissing and trivializing them. Instead, I feel empowered to talk about what I'm going through, not hide it. If I'm feeling this, and feeling alone in it, maybe others are, too.

So, yeah, self-validation is important. It improves self-esteem, self-compassion, and the relationship you have with yourself, as I discussed in chapter 18. One of the qualities that begins to emerge as a relationship strengthens is trust. I want to highlight that by improving how you relate to yourself, self-validation makes it easier for you to trust in your decisions and experiences, allowing you to take input from people without being confused or invalidated by it.

The second point that could use more airtime pertains to external validation. In the book, I model how to validate others and how to validate yourself. I repeatedly normalize the desire for validation from others, but I don't discuss or demonstrate how to obtain it. I worried that focusing on how to receive validation might detract from the emphasis on communicating it, but I've had a change of heart.

It's always been common for us to ask for validation in my house. Last week, when Havana was disappointed to learn she didn't have any friends in her class this school year, I asked if she wanted validation or problem-solving. She said validation and then later reiterated, "Mom, I just want validation," after I suggested we set up playdates with some of the other kids in her class. When I launch into coaching mode with Mat when he's talking about work, he often has to clarify that he's seeking validation, not communication strategies. And when Mat got a judgy look on his face when I said I *needed* to foster another kitten from the shelter, I had to clarify that I was looking for him to validate my need—by Taking Action and going with me—not question my logic.

What's less common is for me to ask for validation from people outside of my immediate family. Like I said, for most of my adult life I've been in the role of caretaker, not care-receiver. Now that cancer has flipped the script, I find myself inundated with texts and messages from people trying to support me, usually by providing data, anecdotes, or other assurances that I'll be okay.

My friends and family are struggling with the same thing I am: fear. And a logical response to fear is to attack the thing that's causing it. What could be more supportive than providing optimistic statistics and success stories of people who overcame the disease that's threatening my life? Such responses are reasonable, and sometimes I'm comforted by them; at other times, the optimism inspires a deep sense of loneliness that paradoxically makes me want to hide. The fact that I'm inconsistent in how I respond from day to day certainly doesn't make things any easier. What has helped is simply asking for validation when I need it. Most everyone who knows me understands this request—at least conceptually—but they might not know how or what to validate. That's fine. There's no harm in providing specifics, as long as it's done gently, not critically. Following are a couple of shameless examples of me seeking external validation:

- I told a family member that I was feeling guilty about all the help I needed and worthless as a result. His immediate reaction was to challenge my emotions: "You can't be serious! You have cancer—go easy on yourself!" I said I appreciated the cheerleading and perspective, but that it would help if he could validate my feelings. He looked confused, so I clarified: "Within a month, I went from being everyone's support system to needing everyone's support. I'm trying to tell myself that it's okay to struggle with the abrupt change and that I don't need to feel bad about feeling bad." He immediately switched gears and started making my case for me by Proposing examples of how I was having to rely on people in ways I hadn't before.
- A well-meaning friend said, "It's just temporary. It will grow back," when I started crying about losing my hair. I gently clarified that what I needed was to feel like my sadness and disappointment were reasonable, not dramatic. She laughed. "I think I'm just trying to talk myself out of crying. Your hair is gorgeous, and it's devastating that you have to lose it!" Side note: I have great hair. Correction to side note: I *had* great hair.

The validation that followed in these situations was not cheapened by my having to ask for it. And as strong as my self-validation practice is, I continue to find that having others see, understand, empathize, and ultimately accept what I'm going through to be restorative. That's putting it mildly. Some days external validation feels like water to parched lips. To be seen by another person, to feel that they accept the reality of what I'm going through—well, there's just something to that. To quote DelGaudio, "It's a fuckin' gift."[1] And desiring that gift doesn't make you weak or needy; it reflects your humanity. To quote renowned social psychologist Mark Leary, "Human beings may differ from other animals most dramatically, not in terms of their tendency to affiliate or interact, but rather in their desire to be accepted by others."[2]

As with any dialectic, the relationship between self and other isn't a matter of either/or, but both/and. You can see the validity in your experiences *and* long for others to see it, too. You can accept yourself *and* be strengthened by the acceptance of others. You can express emotional needs, including the need for validation, *and* have healthy relationships. And while we're on the topic of dialectics, I want to assure all my sisters who might go on to fight breast cancer that you can, in fact, have your boobs removed *and* still have boobs.

If you're reading this epilogue, I'm going to assume you read the introduction and all of the footnotes, too. Again, you are my people. Because it's just us here at the end, I want to thank you for reading my book in its entirety. Regardless of whether you like or agree with my perspective, the combination of Attending (by listening to my words) and Taking Action (by reading what others presumably skipped) validates the work I put into this book. Thank you. I also want to apologize if the epilogue got a little loopy. Chemo brain is a real thing, and I worry these last few pages might sound like they were written by Seth Rogen while he was on a picnic in Amsterdam.

APPENDIX
THE VALIDATION LADDER CHEAT SHEET

Mindfulness Skills	**Attend**
	Show that you're paying attention and listening without judgment.
		• Use the *Big Four*: eye contact, proximity, gesturing, nodding.
		• Play the A Game by asking yourself:
		  - What's a better way to make their point?
		  - Why does it matter (to them)?
		• Ask questions and comment.

	Copy Mirror someone's reaction.	• Mirror their words. • Mirror their ways. • Put words to their ways.
Understanding Skills	**Contextualize** Acknowledge that a person's reaction makes sense in some larger context.	Consider if problematic behavior is valid given: • The past • Misinformation • Disorder
	Equalize Communicate that a person's behavior is equivalent to how others would react.	• Use the Golden Rule approach to foster understanding. • Speak in the first person if you're a peer or authority; use the third person to show deference. • Consider adding the Caroline Qualifier: "and you're handling it better than most."
	Propose Say what you think another person is thinking or feeling.	• Use the A Game, Attending questions, or the Golden Rule approach to generate ideas. • State your idea matter-of-factly or as a suggestion, depending on your level of confidence and the relationship.

Empathy Skills	**Take Action**
	Intervene on someone's behalf.
		They *cannot* intervene themselves:
		• Consider the To Act or Not to Act questions:
		  - Do they have the required resources?
		  - Can and should they learn to do this themselves?
		  - Does the action required go against my values?
		• Ask (for permission) before intervening.
		
		If they *can* Take Action themselves:
		• Remember your intention, and be prepared to back off.

	Emote Express your genuine reaction.	• Use nonverbal behavior. • State thoughts that imply emotions. • Label your feelings using emotion adjectives.
	Disclose Confide shared experiences.	• Focus on shared observations, not the singularity of your thing. • Return the conversation to them after sharing. • Use low-level Disclosures to determine boundaries.

ACKNOWLEDGMENTS

I became obsessed with the *Hamilton* soundtrack while I was writing this manuscript. Havana got pretty into it, too, and would interrupt my focus every now and then by bursting into whatever room I'd holed up in to sing, "Why do you write like you're running out of time?" as loud as she could.

It's a common refrain in the play and one that seemed perfect to tease me with once I began sacrificing my precious weekend hours to write. The weird thing is that I felt privately tortured by the same question. "Why do you write like you're writing out of time?" I wrote on a Post-it note after a particularly compulsive day of writing. Who writes cryptic messages to themselves on Post-it notes? Not me, at least, not historically. Something was up.

I was in a panicked frenzy to complete the book. Those close to me assumed I was under a strict deadline and were surprised to learn that my editor hadn't once pressured me for pages. I think her exact words were, "Delivery dates are only put into contracts to keep them from getting completely out of hands (like years). Don't worry about it." So why did I write like I was running out of time?

I believe in the transformative effects of validation and was excited to get the word out. But that didn't totally explain my behavior. Beneath the surface of my tenacity was the fear that I wouldn't live long enough to complete the book. I realize how dramatic that sounds, but I couldn't shake the sense of foreboding that pressured me to write. I felt a profound sense of relief after finishing the manuscript; not just for having completed it, but because I didn't die in the interim. "Phew," I remember thinking, "my fear of death wasn't a premonition!" Diligent epilogue readers know that the relief didn't last long. Within a week of completing the book, I was diagnosed with breast cancer. The disease was invasive and aggressive and had spread through my lymph nodes.

Although I was done writing, I still had a fair amount of work ahead of me to prepare the manuscript for publication. Once again, I worried that I was running out of time, only now it appeared my fear might be valid.

The thing about cancer is that it puts things in perspective. I developed an infection after my double mastectomy that could have been life-threatening; I experienced cardiac distress after my third chemotherapy and was told I was either suffering from severe sepsis or heart failure (it turned out to be neither). Death felt imminent, and once it became clear that I might really be running out of time, I didn't want to write anymore. I didn't want to do anything except be around my family. Unless they *were* around, then I wanted to be alone to vomit, and sleep, and have diarrhea in solitude.

The other thing about cancer is that it has a way of revealing people's character. When folks hear you have cancer, they almost always respond with sympathy and concern—neither of which is particularly telling. The character-revealing moments are reflected in the ways people Take Action, particularly when at a cost to themselves. The team that was assembled to work on this book was made up of exceptionally talented individuals. That much was clear (and intimidating) to me from the beginning, but I didn't realize the true character of many of these folks until cancer revealed them to me.

It is these "characters" that I'd like to acknowledge first because, without them, I don't know if I'd have seen this book through to publication. To Caroline Sutton (me from the future), thank you for dissolving my insecurities with laughter, as you so often did, and for being the light that helped me find my way through so many dark tunnels. To the fine folks at Avery, who, despite noting that publishing dates are only used to keep manuscripts from getting pushed out for years, responded to the news of my diagnosis by extending my publication date by years in case I needed it. To Lucia Watson, who stepped up when I was down and out from radiation to help move the manuscript through editing without ever making me feel pressured. To my agent, Giles Anderson, who believed first in my ability to write this book, and later that cancer would slow, but not stop me, from publishing it. To my longtime assistant, Kyla Krontz, who did everything shy of seeing my clients and becoming a ghostwriter to keep me afloat. And to Geraldine Rodriguez, who embodied the validation and selflessness her mother championed.

To my judgmental cat, who was so pissed when she heard the doctor say I'd need to start chemotherapy that she died the next day, and to the kittens who tried to fill her enormous cat shoes by eating everything in sight including, and I'm not kidding, an entire loaf of bread. And to my friends and family, thank you for continuing to reach out with love and support, even though I so often failed to reinforce you with a response. You defy the laws of behaviorism.

I'd also like to acknowledge those who influenced me well before all of this breast-cancer business. To Jackie Gollan, Zach Rosenthal, Jennifer Sayrs, Marsha Linehan, Jianhu Shifu, and the late Clive Robins, who were all instrumental in shaping my work—and life, for that matter. To my colleagues over the years—who were so good at validation, they couldn't help but become friends—Betsy Holmberg, Katrina Blomquist, Dorian Hunter, Jared Michonski, Julia Hitch, Clara Doctolero, Angela Davis, Sanno Zack, Soo Uhm, Julie Leader, Hal Lynne Micali, Samantha Fordwood, Jeanne Jakob, Jennifer Nam, Molly Walsh, and the late Ayelet Kattan. To my editorial glam squad, with special thanks to Andrea St. Aubin, Christy Wagner, Maria Tilden, and my brother, Jef, who is the real writer in our family.

Last, by intention and for emphasis, to Mat and Havana. Mat, in addition to letting me share secret recordings of our conversations with the world, you read every page I wrote, emptied my breast drains after surgery, edited chapters at all hours of the day and night, registered Havana for summer camps, pirated a copy of Adobe Illustrator when I was in a pinch, and Took Action in countless ways while I wrote like I was running out of time, and in the dark days that followed when we feared I might actually be. I'm reminded of something Caroline Sutton said to me when I was singing your praises: "Doesn't being married to a nice guy make you feel like a total bitch sometimes?" It does, Mat, it really does.

Havana, this work has been my effort to "make the world safe and sound for yooooooooou." I dedicate it to you, Mu. P.S. I'm sorry my book on validation is getting published first; yours has way better illustrations.

NOTES

INTRODUCTION

1. **REDUCING OPIOID USE:** Marsha M. Linehan et al., "Dialectical Behavior Therapy versus Comprehensive Validation Therapy plus 12-Step for the Treatment of Opioid Dependent Women Meeting Criteria for Borderline Personality Disorder," *Drug and Alcohol Dependence* 67, no. 1 (June 1, 2002): 13–26, https://doi.org/10.1016/s0376-8716(02)00011-x.

CHAPTER 1: VALIDATION—PSYCHOLOGY'S BEST-KEPT SECRET

1. **IT'S TRUE THAT EXPERTS IN CLINICAL PSYCHOLOGY:** James A. Blumenthal et al., "Exercise and Pharmacotherapy in the Treatment of Major Depressive Disorder," *Psychosomatic Medicine* 69, no. 7 (September 1, 2007): 587–96, https://doi.org/10.1097/psy.0b013e318148c19a.

2. **IN PEOPLE WITH THESE CONDITIONS:** Marsha M. Linehan et al., "Cognitive-Behavioral Treatment of Chronically Parasuicidal Borderline Patients," *Archives of General Psychiatry* 48, no. 12 (December 1, 1991): 1060–64, https://doi.org/10.1001/archpsyc.1991.01810360024003; Shuyan Chen et al., "Effects of Dialectical Behaviour Therapy on Reducing Self-Harming Behaviours and Negative Emotions in Patients with Borderline Personality Disorder: A Meta-Analysis," *Journal of Psychiatric and Mental Health Nursing* 28, no. 6 (December 1, 2021): 1128–39, https://doi.org/10.1111/jpm .12797.

3. **SEE THE MERIT OF THIS PERSPECTIVE:** Ethan H. Mereish, Conall O'Cleirigh, and Judith Bradford, "Interrelationships Between LGBT-Based Victimization, Suicide, and Substance Use Problems in a Diverse Sample of Sexual and Gender Minorities," *Psychology, Health & Medicine* 19, no. 1 (March 27, 2013): 1–13, https://doi.org/10.1080/13548506.2013.780129; Kristen Clements-Nolle et al., "HIV Prevalence, Risk Behaviors, Health Care Use, and Mental Health Status of Transgender Persons: Implications for Public Health Intervention," *American Journal of Public Health* 91, no. 6 (June 1, 2001): 915–21, https://doi.org/10.2105/ajph.91.6.915; Ann C. Haas et al., "Suicide and Suicide Risk in Lesbian, Gay, Bisexual, and Transgender Populations: Review and Recommendations," *Journal of*

Homosexuality 58, no. 1 (December 30, 2010): 10–51, https://doi.org/10
.1080/00918369.2011.534038.

4. **"IMPORTANCE OF VALIDATION IN DBT":** Marsha M. Linehan, "Validation and Psychotherapy," in *Empathy Reconsidered: New Directions in Psychotherapy*, eds. A. C. Bohart and L. S. Greenberg (Washington, DC: American Psychological Association, 1997), 355, https://doi.org/10.1037/10226-016.

5. **RECURRENT DEPRESSION:** Walter E. B. Sipe and Stuart J. Eisendrath, "Mindfulness-Based Cognitive Therapy for Treatment-Resistant Depression," in *Mindfulness-Based Treatment Approaches: Clinician's Guide to Evidence Base and Applications*, 2nd ed., ed. Ruth Ware (Waltham, MA: Academic Press, 2014), 61–76.

6. **BORDERLINE PERSONALITY DISORDER:** Alec L. Miller, "Introduction to a Special Issue Dialectical Behavior Therapy: Evolution and Adaptations in the 21st Century," *American Journal of Psychotherapy* 69, no. 2 (January 1, 2015): 91–95, https://doi.org/10.1176/appi.psychotherapy.2015.69.2.91.

7. **I SAW A VIDEO:** Weight Watchers, "Oprah's 2020 Vision Tour Visionaries: Lady Gaga Interview," YouTube, January 9, 2020, https://www.youtube .com/watch?v=f8iNYY7YV04.

8. **"RADICAL ACCEPTANCE," THE DBT SKILL:** Marsha M. Linehan, *DBT Skills Training Handouts and Worksheets*, 2nd ed., "Distress Tolerance Handout 11: Radical Acceptance" (New York: Guilford Publications, 2014).

9. **FOLLOWING THE SUCCESS OF MINDFULNESS-BASED STRESS REDUCTION (MBSR):** Jon Kabat-Zinn, *Full Catastrophe Living: Using the Wisdom of Your Body and Mind to Face Stress, Pain, and Illness* (New York: Bantam Books, an imprint of Random House, 1990).

10. **IMPROVED CONDITIONS AS DIVERSE AS CHRONIC PAIN:** Jon Kabat-Zinn, "An Outpatient Program in Behavioral Medicine for Chronic Pain Patients Based on the Practice of Mindfulness Meditation: Theoretical Considerations and Preliminary Results," *General Hospital Psychiatry* 4, no. 1 (April 1, 1982): 33–47, https://doi.org/10.1016/0163-8343(82)90026-3; Jon Kabat-Zinn, Leslie Lipworth, and Robert G. Burney, "The Clinical Use of Mindfulness Meditation for the Self-Regulation of Chronic Pain," *Journal of Behavioral Medicine* 8, no. 2 (June 1, 1985): 163–90, https://doi.org/10.1007/bf00845519.

11. **AND ANXIETY:** Jon Kabat-Zinn et al., "Effectiveness of a Meditation-Based Stress Reduction Program in the Treatment of Anxiety Disorders," *American Journal of Psychiatry* 149, no. 7 (July 1, 1992): 936–43, https://doi.org/10 .1176/ajp.149.7.936.

12. **HE DEFINED MINDFULNESS AS:** Jon Kabat-Zinn, *Wherever You Go, There You Are: Mindfulness Meditation in Everyday Life* (New York: Hyperion, 2005), 4; Shian-Ling Keng, Moria J. Smoski, and Clive J. Robins, "Effects of Mindfulness on Psychological Health: A Review of Empirical Studies," *Clinical Psychology Review* 31, no. 6 (August 1, 2011): 1041–56, https://doi.org/10.1016 /j.cpr.2011.04.006.

13. **"VALIDATION HAS NOTHING TO DO WITH SOCIAL DESIRABILITY"**: Linehan, "Validation and Psychotherapy," 358.

14. **AMONG THOSE TAUGHT TO CLIENTS**: Linehan, *DBT Skills Training*, 110–11.

15. **BETTER COMMUNICATE WITH YOUR PARTNER**: Scott D. Stanley, Howard J. Markman, and Susan L. Blumberg, "The Speaker/Listener Technique," *The Family Journal* 5, no. 1 (January 1, 1997): 82–83, https://doi.org/10.1177/1066480797051013.

16. **TO HELP YOU EFFECTIVELY MITIGATE CONFLICTS**: Kerry Patterson et al., *Crucial Conversations Tools for Talking When Stakes Are High*, 2nd ed. (New York: McGraw Hill Professional, 2011), 164.

17. **"MIRRORING"**: Tom Bunn, "Megaphone Parenting Can't Meet a Child's Need for Mirroring," *Psychology Today*, September 16, 2019, https://www.psychologytoday.com/us/blog/conquer-fear-flying/201909/megaphone-parenting-cant-meet-childs-need-mirroring.

18. **". . . AND IT'S UP TO YOU TO MAKE THAT HAPPEN"**: The White House, Office of the Press Secretary, *Remarks of President Barack Obama at Student Roundtable in Istanbul*, April 7, 2009, https://obamawhitehouse.archives.gov/reality check/the-press-office/remarks-president-barack-obama-student -roundtable-istanbul.

CHAPTER 2: A CURE FOR ALL—WHY YOU SHOULD DROP EVERYTHING AND LEARN TO VALIDATE

1. *INTIMACY, AND PSYCHOLOGICAL SAFETY*: Jonathan W. Kanter et al., "An Integrative Contextual Behavioral Model of Intimate Relations," *Journal of Contextual Behavioral Science* 18 (October 1, 2020): 75–91, https://doi.org/10.1016/j.jcbs.2020.09.001; Yan Ruan et al., "Can I Tell You How I Feel? Perceived Partner Responsiveness Encourages Emotional Expression," *Emotion* 20, no. 3 (April 1, 2020): 329–42, https://doi.org/10.1037/emo0000650.

2. **RESEARCH HAS CONSISTENTLY SHOWN**: Shelly L. Gable, Gian C. Gonzaga, and Amy Strachman, "Will You Be There for Me When Things Go Right? Supportive Responses to Positive Event Disclosures," *Journal of Personality and Social Psychology* 91, no. 5 (November 1, 2006): 904–17, https://doi.org/10.1037/0022-3514.91.5.904; Amy Canevello and Jennifer Crocker, "Creating Good Relationships: Responsiveness, Relationship Quality, and Interpersonal Goals," *Journal of Personality and Social Psychology* 99, no. 1 (July 1, 2010): 78–106, https://doi.org/10.1037/a0018186; Kanter et al., "An Integrative Contextual Behavioral Model."

3. **FIFTEEN CIGARETTES A DAY**: Julianne Holt-Lunstad, Timothy W. Smith, and J. Bradley Layton, "Social Relationships and Mortality Risk: A Meta-Analytic Review," *PLOS Medicine* 7, no. 7 (July 27, 2010): e1000316, https://doi.org/10.1371/journal.pmed.1000316.

4. **PROBABILITY OF SURVIVING BY 50 PERCENT**: Holt-Lunstad, Smith, and Layton, "Social Relationships and Mortality Risk."

5. **IN A CLEVER STUDY:** Steven J. Linton et al., "Painfully Reassuring? The Effects of Validation on Emotions and Adherence in a Pain Test," *European Journal of Pain* 16, no. 4 (April 1, 2012): 592–99, https://doi.org/10.1016/j.ejpain.2011.07.011.

6. **THEIR EXTENSIVE RESEARCH SHOWS:** Laurence Alison and Emily Alison. "Revenge versus Rapport: Interrogation, Terrorism, and Torture," *American Psychologist* 72, no. 3 (April 1, 2017): 266–77, https://doi.org/10.1037/amp0000064.

7. **RAPPORT IS MORE OR LESS SYNONYMOUS WITH VALIDATION:** Laurence Alison and Emily Alison, "Revenge versus Rapport," 270.

8. **STUDIES HAVE CONCLUSIVELY SHOWN:** Laurence Alison et al., "The Efficacy of Rapport-Based Techniques for Minimizing Counter-Interrogation Tactics Amongst a Field Sample of Terrorists," *Psychology, Public Policy and Law* 20, no. 4 (November 1, 2014): 421–30, https://doi.org/10.1037/law0000021; Laurence Alison et al., "Why Tough Tactics Fail and Rapport Gets Results: Observing Rapport-Based Interpersonal Techniques (ORBIT) to Generate Useful Information from Terrorists," *Psychology, Public Policy and Law* 19, no. 4 (November 1, 2013): 411–31, https://doi.org/10.1037/a0034564.

9. **VALIDATION HAS BEEN SHOWN TO DECREASE DEFENSIVENESS:** For a review of the research on validation and customer satisfaction, see Carol M. Werner et al., "Clinical Validation and Cognitive Elaboration: Signs That Encourage Sustained Recycling," *Basic and Applied Social Psychology* 24, no. 3 (September 1, 2002): 185–203, https://doi.org/10.1207/s15324834basp2403_2.

10. **VALIDATION TEMPERS THIS RESPONSE:** Alan E. Fruzzetti and John M. Worrall, "Accurate Expression and Validating Responses: A Transactional Model for Understanding Individual and Relationship Distress," in *Support Processes in Intimate Relationships*, eds. Kieran T. Sullivan and Joanne Davila (online ed: Oxford Academic, 2010), 121–50, https://doi.org/10.1093/acprof:oso/9780195380170.003.0005.

11. **VALIDATING PEOPLE IN HIGHLY STRESSFUL SITUATIONS:** Chad E. Shenk and Alan E. Fruzzetti, "The Impact of Validating and Invalidating Responses on Emotional Reactivity," *Journal of Social and Clinical Psychology* 30, no. 2 (February 22, 2011): 163–83, https://doi.org/10.1521/jscp.2011.30.2.163.

12. **INVALIDATION HAS PROVEN TO HAVE THE OPPOSITE EFFECT:** Maddy Greville-Harris et al., "The Power of Invalidating Communication: Receiving Invalidating Feedback Predicts Threat-Related Emotional, Physiological, and Social Responses," *Journal of Social and Clinical Psychology* 35, no. 6 (June 1, 2016): 471–93, https://doi.org/10.1521/jscp.2016.35.6.471.

13. **RESEARCH ON INTIMATE AND SIBLING RELATIONSHIPS:** Nina Howe et al., "Siblings as Confidants: Emotional Understanding, Relationship Warmth, and Sibling Self-Disclosure," *Social Development* 10, no. 4 (November 1, 2001): 439–54, https://doi.org/10.1111/1467-9507.00174; Lawrence R. Wheeless and Janis Grotz, "The Measurement of Trust and Its Relationship to

Self-Disclosure," *Human Communication Research* 3, no. 3 (March 1, 1977): 250–57, https://doi.org/10.1111/j.1468-2958.1977.tb00523.x; Kristin Behfar, Matthew A. Cronin, and Kimberly McCarthy, "Realizing the Upside of Venting: The Role of the 'Challenger Listener,'" *Academy of Management Discoveries* 6, no. 4 (December 1, 2020): 609–30, https://doi.org/10.5465/amd.2018.0066.

14. **THESE OUTCOMES ARE CONSISTENT WITH RESEARCH:** Christina Gamache Martin, Hyoun Woo Kim, and Jennifer J. Freyd, "In the Spirit of Full Disclosure: Maternal Distress, Emotion Validation, and Adolescent Disclosure of Distressing Experiences," *Emotion* 18, no. 3 (September 4, 2017): 400–11, https://doi.org/10.1037/emo0000363.

15. **HOLD TRUE EVEN FOR STRANGERS:** Kevin G. Haworth et al., "Reinforcement Matters: A Preliminary, Laboratory-Based Component-Process Analysis of Functional Analytic Psychotherapy's Model of Social Connection," *Journal of Contextual Behavioral Science* 4, no. 4 (October 1, 2015): 281–91, https://doi.org/10.1016/j.jcbs.2015.08.003.

16. **A STUDY AT COLUMBIA UNIVERSITY:** Vincent Guilamo-Ramos, "Dominican and Puerto Rican Mother-Adolescent Communication: Maternal Self-Disclosure and Youth Risk Intentions," *Hispanic Journal of Behavioral Sciences* 32, no. 2 (May 1, 2010): 197–215, https://doi.org/10.1177/0739986310361594.

17. **IN AN EVEN MORE SHOCKING STUDY:** Nicole M. Froidevaux et al., "The Link Between Adversity and Dating Violence Among Adolescents Hospitalized for Psychiatric Treatment: Parental Emotion Validation as a Candidate Protective Factor," *Journal of Interpersonal Violence* 37, no. 5–6 (March 1, 2022): NP3492–NP 3527, https://doi.org/10.1177/0886260520926323.

18. **NEUROIMAGING RESEARCH HAS SHOWN:** Sylvia A. Morelli, Jared B. Torre, and Naomi I. Eisenberger, "The Neural Bases of Feeling Understood and Not Understood," *Social Cognitive and Affective Neuroscience* 9, no. 12 (December 1, 2014): 1890–96, https://doi.org/10.1093/scan/nst191.

19. **VERBAL REWARDS HAVE PROVEN:** Konstanze Albrecht et al., "The Brain Correlates of the Effects of Monetary and Verbal Rewards on Intrinsic Motivation," *Frontiers in Neuroscience* 8 (September 18, 2014), https://doi.org/10.3389/fnins.2014.00303.

20. **IN *THE MINDFUL SELF-COMPASSION WORKBOOK*:** Kristin Neff and Christopher Germer, *The Mindful Self-Compassion Workbook: A Proven Way to Accept Yourself, Build Inner Strength, and Thrive* (New York: Guilford Press, 2018), 9.

21. **SYMPTOMS OF DEPRESSION, ANXIETY:** Phan Y. Hong and David A. Lishner, "General Invalidation and Trauma-Specific Invalidation as Predictors of Personality and Subclinical Psychopathology," *Personality and Individual Differences* 89 (January 1, 2016): 211–16, https://doi.org/10.1016/j.paid.2015.10.016.

22. **A 2021 STUDY PUBLISHED BY THE AMERICAN PSYCHOLOGICAL ASSOCIATION:** Marisa G. Franco, Myles I. Durkee, and Stacey E. McElroy-Heltzel,

"Discrimination Comes in Layers: Dimensions of Discrimination and Mental Health for Multiracial People," *Cultural Diversity and Ethnic Minority Psychology* 27, no. 3 (May 3, 2021): 343–53, https://doi.org/10.1037/cdp0000441.

23. **IDENTITY INVALIDATION HAS BEEN REPORTED:** Brian A. Feinstein et al., "A Qualitative Examination of Bisexual+ Identity Invalidation and Its Consequences for Wellbeing, Identity, and Relationships," *Journal of Bisexuality* 19, no. 4 (October 2, 2019): 461–82, https://doi.org/10.1080/15299716.2019.1671295; Kelly E. Johnson et al., "Invalidation Experiences and Protective Factors Among Non-Binary Adolescents," *Journal of Adolescent Health*, February 1, 2019, https://doi.org/10.1016/j.jadohealth.2018.10.021.

24. **A UNIQUE CONTRIBUTOR TO GENDER INEQUALITY:** Michael W. Salter, "Invalidation: A Neglected Dimension of Gender-Based Violence and Inequality," *International Journal for Crime, Justice and Social Democracy* 1, no. 1 (November 5, 2012): 3–13, https://doi.org/10.5204/ijcjsd.v1i1.73.

25. **FROM FAMILY MEMBERS:** Sara Edlund et al., "I See You're in Pain—The Effects of Partner Validation on Emotions in People with Chronic Pain," *Scandinavian Journal of Pain* 6, no. 1 (January 1, 2015): 16–21, https://doi.org/10.1016/j.sjpain.2014.07.003.

26. **TO STUDENTS:** Steven J. Linton et al., "Can Training in Empathetic Validation Improve Medical Students' Communication with Patients Suffering Pain? A Test of Concept," *Pain Reports* 2, no. 3 (April 30, 2017): e600, https://doi.org/10.1097/pr9.0000000000000600.

27. **AND DOCTORS:** Riikka Holopainen et al., "Physiotherapists' Validating and Invalidating Communication Before and After Participating in Brief Cognitive Functional Therapy Training. Test of Concept Study," *Advances in Physiotherapy* 25, no. 2 (September 23, 2021): 1–7, https://doi.org/10.1080/21679169.2021.1967446.

28. **SIGNIFICANT CHANGES HAVE BEEN REPORTED:** Linton et al., "Training in Empathetic Validation."

29. **IN ONE EXPERIMENT AFTER ONLY FORTY-FIVE MINUTES:** Edlund et al., "I See You're in Pain."

CHAPTER 3: WHAT IT MEANS TO BE SEEN—VALIDATION DEFINED

1. **YOU CAN THANK THE NEGATIVITY BIAS FOR THAT:** Paul Rozin and Edward B. Royzman, "Negativity Bias, Negativity Dominance, and Contagion," *Personality and Social Psychology Review* 5, no. 4 (November 1, 2001): 296–320, https://doi.org/10.1207/s15327957pspr0504_2.

CHAPTER 4: VALIDATION AND THE ART OF SUFFERING—ONE LAST REASON TO DROP EVERYTHING AND LEARN TO VALIDATE

1. **AS THE LATE, GREAT CARL ROGERS SAID:** Carl R. Rogers, *Client-Centered Therapy: Its Current Practice, Implications and Theory*, 70th anniversary ed. (London: Constable & Robinson Ltd, 2021), 230.

2. **IN 1957, HE PUBLISHED A NOW-LEGENDARY PAPER:** Carl R. Rogers, "The Necessary and Sufficient Conditions of Therapeutic Personality Change," *Journal of Consulting Psychology* 21, no. 2 (1957): 95–103, https://doi.org /10.1037/h0045357.

3. **ROGERS REJECTED THE VIEWS OF BEHAVIORISTS:** Carl R. Rogers, "Toward a Science of the Person," *Journal of Humanistic Psychology* 3, no. 2 (April 1, 1963): 72–92, https://doi.org/10.1177/002216786300300208.

4. **HE ALSO TOOK ISSUE WITH THE HOLIER-THAN-THOU:** Eugene T. Gendlin, "Obituary: Carl Rogers (1902–1987)," *American Psychologist* 43, no. 2 (February 1, 1988): 127–28, https://doi.org/10.1037/h0091937; Barry A. Farber and Erin M. Doolin, "Positive Regard and Affirmation," in *Psychotherapy Relationships That Work: Evidence-Based Responsiveness*, 2nd ed., ed. John C. Norcross (New York: Oxford University Press, 2011): 171.

5. **DISAPPOINTED BY THE STATE OF HIS FIELD:** David Lester, "Active Listening," in *Crisis Intervention and Counseling by Telephone and Internet*, eds. David Lester and James Rogers (Springfield, IL: Charles C. Thomas Publisher, 2012), 94.

6. **HE CAUTIONED THERAPISTS:** Carl R. Rogers, "Significant Aspects of Client-Centered Therapy," *American Psychologist* 1, no. 10 (January 1, 1946): 415–22, https://doi.org/10.1037/h0060866.

7. **"'YOU'RE NOT LISTENING TO ME':** Marsha M. Linehan, *Building a Life Worth Living: A Memoir* (New York: Random House, 2020), 214.

8. **"'WHAT? YOU'RE NOT GOING TO HELP ME?':** Linehan, *Building A Life Worth Living*, 215.

9. **LINEHAN TOOK A HIATUS:** BorderlineNotes, "Marsha Linehan—How She Learned Radical Acceptance," YouTube, April 14, 2017, https://www .youtube.com/watch?v=OTG7YEWkJFI&t=11s.

10. **THE "DIALECTICAL" IN DIALECTICAL BEHAVIOR THERAPY:** Linehan, *Building A Life Worth Living*, 226.

11. **DBT'S LEVELS OF VALIDATION:** Linehan, *DBT Skills Training*, "Interpersonal Effectiveness Handout 18: A 'How To' Guide to Validation."

12. **ACCORDING TO LINEHAN, EACH LEVEL IS MORE COMPLETE:** Marsha M. Linehan, "Validation and Psychotherapy," in *Empathy Reconsidered: New Directions in Psychotherapy*, eds. A. C. Bohart and L. S. Greenberg (Washington, DC: American Psychological Association, 1997), 360, https://doi. org/10.1037/10226-016.

13. **NO MUD, NO FLOWERS:** Thich Nhat Hanh, *No Mud, No Lotus: The Art of Transforming Suffering* (Berkeley: Parallax Press, 2014).

14. **"DESPAIR IS SUFFERING WITHOUT MEANING":** Viktor Emil Frankl, *The Unconscious God* (New York: Pocket Books, 1975), 137.

15. **IN THE WORDS OF THICH NHAT HANH:** Hanh, *No Mud, No Lotus*, 10.

16. **"EPIDEMIC OF LONELINESS":** Vivek Murthy, "Work and the Loneliness Epidemic," *Harvard Business Review*, November 8, 2022, https://hbr.org/2017 /09/work-and-the-loneliness-epidemic.

CHAPTER 6: ATTEND—THE GAME ALL GOOD LISTENERS PLAY

1. **DELGAUDIO SAID IN AN INTERVIEW WITH GQ MAGAZINE:** Sam Schube, "Derek DelGaudio's Genre-Bending Magic Show Will Make You Feel Things," *GQ*, July 16, 2018, https://www.gq.com/story/derek-delgaudio-magician -profile.

2. **IN PHYSICS, THE "OBSERVER EFFECT":** Eric Dent, "The Observation, Inquiry, and Measurement Challenges Surfaced by Complexity Theory," in *Managing the Complex: Philosophy, Theory and Practice*, ed. Kurt Richardson (Charlotte, NC: Information Age Publishers, 2004).

3. **IN WHAT CAME TO BE KNOWN AS THE HAWTHORNE EFFECT:** Helen Parsons, "What Happened at Hawthorne?" *Science* 183, no. 4128 (March 8, 1974): 922–32, https://doi.org/10.1126/science.183.4128.922.

4. **"I FELL IN LOVE WITH HER":** *My Octopus Teacher*, directed by James Reed and Pippa Ehlrich (Off the Fence and The Sea Change Project, 2020), Netflix.

5. **ACADEMY AWARD FOR BEST DOCUMENTARY FEATURE:** "The 93rd Academy Awards | 2021," Oscars.org, Academy of Motion Picture Arts and Sciences, accessed May 2, 2023, https://www.oscars.org/oscars/ceremonies /2021.

6. **THEY REFER TO THESE NONVERBALS AS "IMMEDIACY BEHAVIORS,":** Janis F. Andersen, Peter A. Andersen, and Arthur D. Jensen, "The Measurement of Nonverbal Immediacy," *Journal of Applied Communication Research* 7, no. 2 (November 1, 1979): 153–80, https://doi.org/10.1080/00909887909365204.

7. **EYE CONTACT, 2. PROXIMITY, 3. GESTURING, 4. NODDING:** Janis Andersen, Peter Andersen, and Jensen, "Measurement of Nonverbal Immediacy"; Laura K. Guerrero, "Conceptualizing and Operationalizing Nonverbal Immediacy," in *Researching Interactive Communication Behavior: A Sourcebook of Methods and Measures*, eds. C. Arthur VanLear and Daniel J. Canary (Thousand Oaks, CA: SAGE Publications Inc., 2017), 61–75.

CHAPTER 7: COPY—HOW TO CONNECT WITH ANYONE

1. **POSITIVELY AFFECTS HOW THEY FEEL:** Mariëlle Stel and Roos Vonk, "Mimicry in Social Interaction: Benefits for Mimickers, Mimickees, and Their Interaction," *British Journal of Psychology* 101, no. 2 (May 1, 2010): 311–13, https://doi.org/10.1348/000712609x465424; Tanya L. Chartrand and John A. Bargh, "The Chameleon Effect: The Perception–Behavior Link and Social Interaction," *Journal of Personality and Social Psychology* 76, no. 6 (January 1, 1999): 893–910, https://doi.org/10.1037/0022-3514.76.6.893.

2. **IN PERHAPS THE MOST FAMOUS STUDY ON COPYING:** Rick B. van Baaren et al., "Mimicry for Money: Behavioral Consequences of Imitation," *Journal of Experimental Social Psychology* 39, no. 4 (July 1, 2003): 393–98, https://doi .org/10.1016/s0022-1031(03)00014-3.

3. **SIMILAR RESULTS WERE REPORTED:** Rick B. van Baaren et al., "Mimicry and

Prosocial Behavior," *Psychological Science* 15, no. 1 (January 1, 2004): 71–74, https://doi.org/10.1111/j.0963-7214.2004.01501012.x.

4. **BOTH REPORT MORE CONNECTION AND A STRONGER:** Stel and Vonk, "Mimicry in Social Interaction."

5. **IMPLICIT RACISM REFERS TO:** Bailey Maryfield, "Implicit Racial Bias," Justice Research and Statistics Association, December 2018, https://api .semanticscholar.org/CorpusID:231601864.

6. **SHOWED AN IMPLICIT BIAS AGAINST BLACK PEOPLE:** Michael Inzlicht, Jennifer N. Gutsell, and Lisa Legault, "Mimicry Reduces Racial Prejudice," *Journal of Experimental Social Psychology* 48, no. 1 (January 1, 2012): 361–65, https://doi.org/10.1016/j.jesp.2011.06.007.

7. **IN THE MOST INGENIOUS USE OF THE XBOX 360:** Ron Tamborini et al., "The Effect of Behavioral Synchrony with Black or White Virtual Agents on Outgroup Trust," *Computers in Human Behavior* 83 (June 1, 2018): 176–83, https://doi.org/10.1016/j.chb.2018.01.037.

8. **REDUCES VICTIM-BLAMING:** Mariëlle Stel, Kees van den Bos, and Michèlle Bal, "On Mimicry and the Psychology of the Belief in a Just World: Imitating the Behaviors of Others Reduces the Blaming of Innocent Victims," *Social Justice Research* 25, no. 1 (February 29, 2012): 14–24, https://doi.org /10.1007/s11211-012-0150-2.

9. **COMPELS PEOPLE TO GIVE MORE TO CHARITY:** Mariëlle Stel, Rick B. van Baaren, and Roos Vonk, "Effects of Mimicking: Acting Prosocially by Being Emotionally Moved," *European Journal of Social Psychology* 38, no. 6 (September 1, 2008): 965–76, https://doi.org/10.1002/ejsp.472.

10. **TOWARD CITIZENS ON OPPOSITE SIDES OF A WAR:** Béatrice S. Hasler et al., "Virtual Peacemakers: Mimicry Increases Empathy in Simulated Contact with Virtual Outgroup Members," *Cyberpsychology, Behavior, and Social Networking* 17, no. 12 (December 9, 2014): 766–71, https://doi.org/10.1089 /cyber.2014.0213.

11. **IN THE REALM OF DATING:** Nicolas Guéguen, "Mimicry and Seduction: An Evaluation in a Courtship Context," *Social Influence* 4, no. 4 (September 14, 2009): 249–55, https://doi.org/10.1080/15534510802628173.

12. **SOMETIMES REFERRED TO AS THE CHAMELEON EFFECT:** Tanya L. Chartrand and John A. Bargh, "The Chameleon Effect: The Perception–Behavior Link and Social Interaction," *Journal of Personality and Social Psychology* 76, no. 6 (January 1, 1999): 893–910, https://doi.org/10.1037/0022-3514.76.6 .893; Jessica L. Lakin et al., "The Chameleon Effect as Social Glue: Evidence for the Evolutionary Significance of Nonconscious Mimicry," *Journal of Nonverbal Behavior* 27, no. 3 (September 1, 2003): 145–62, https://doi .org/10.1023/a:1025389814290.

13. **STUDIES OF BABIES SHOW:** Andrew N. Meltzoff and M. Keith Moore, "Imitation in Newborn Infants: Exploring the Range of Gestures Imitated and the Underlying Mechanisms," *Developmental Psychology* 25, no. 6 (November 1, 1989): 954–62, https://doi.org/10.1037/0012-1649.25.6.954; Jeannette

M. Haviland and Michelle Mary Lelwica, "The Induced Affect Response: 10-Week-Old Infants' Responses to Three Emotion Expressions," *Developmental Psychology* 23, no. 1 (January 1, 1987): 97–104, https://doi.org /10.1037/0012-1649.23.1.97.

14. **TO BUILD A TRIBE, YOU MUST BE ABLE TO UNDERSTAND AND EMPATHIZE:** For a review of the developmental research on Copying and Empathy, see Stel and Vonk, "Mimicry in Social Interaction."

15. **BY WAY OF THIS TRUSTY LITTLE FEEDBACK LOOP:** Ursula Hess et al., "The Facilitative Effect of Facial Expression on the Self-Generation of Emotion," *International Journal of Psychophysiology* 12, no. 3 (May 1, 1992): 251–65, https://doi.org/10.1016/0167-8760(92)90064-i; Daniel H. McIntosh, "Facial Feedback Hypotheses: Evidence, Implications, and Directions," *Motivation and Emotion* 20, no. 2 (June 1, 1996): 121–47, https://doi.org/10.1007 /bf02253868; Mariëlle Stel and Kees van den Bos, "Mimicry as a Tool for Understanding the Emotions of Other," in *Proceedings of Measuring Behavior*, eds. Andrew Spink et al. (Eindhoven, The Netherlands: Noldus Information Technology, 2010), 114–17.

16. **COPYING LEADS *BOTH* THE COPIER AND THE PERSON BEING COPIED:** Stel and Vonk, "Mimicry in Social Interaction."

17. .**COPY PEOPLE WHO ARE ATTRACTIVE:** Barbara Müller et al., "Empathy Is a Beautiful Thing: Empathy Predicts Imitation Only for Attractive Others," *Scandinavian Journal of Psychology* 54, no. 5 (October 1, 2013): 401–6, https://doi.org/10.1111/sjop.12060; Jie Shen et al., "The Influence of Facial Attractiveness and Personal Characteristics on Imitation," *Journal of Social Psychology* 163, no. 1 (2023): 94–106.

18. **IN POSITIONS OF POWER:** Clara M. Cheng and Tanya L. Chartrand, "Self-Monitoring Without Awareness: Using Mimicry as a Nonconscious Affiliation Strategy," *Journal of Personality and Social Psychology* 85, no. 6 (December 1, 2003): 1170–79, https://doi.org/10.1037/0022-3514.85.6.1170.

19. **COPYING PEOPLE IS NO LESS EFFECTIVE WHEN:** Nobuyuki Nishitani, Sari Avikainen, and Riitta Hari, "Abnormal Imitation-Related Cortical Activation Sequences in Asperger's Syndrome," *Annals of Neurology* 55, no. 4 (April 1, 2004): 558–62, https://doi.org/10.1002/ana.20031.

20. **WITH MORE THAN 90 PERCENT ACCURACY:** John M. Gottman et al., "Predicting Marital Happiness and Stability from Newlywed Interactions," *Journal of Marriage and Family* 60, no. 1 (February 1, 1998): 5, https://doi.org /10.2307/353438; John M. Gottman, *What Predicts Divorce?: The Relationship Between Marital Processes and Marital Outcomes* (Hillsdale, NJ: Lawrence Erlbaum Associates, 1994).

21. **PARTNERS WHO SIMPLY READ HIS BOOK:** Julia C. Babcock et al., "A Component Analysis of a Brief Psycho-Educational Couples' Workshop: One-Year Follow-up Results," *Journal of Family Therapy* 35, no. 3 (August 1, 2013): 252–80, https://doi.org/10.1111/1467-6427.12017.

22. **I ENCOUNTERED THE GOTTMAN-RAPOPORT INTERVENTION:** John M. Gottman and Julie Schwartz Gottman, *Gottman Rapoport Intervention* (The Gottman Institute, 2015).

CHAPTER 8: CONTEXTUALIZE—SOLVING FOR WHY

1. **JENNY LAWSON, CONTEXTUALIZING:** Jenny Lawson, "Our Stories Set Us Free," TEDx SanAntonio, January 8, 2020, https://www.ted.com/talks/jenny _lawson_our_stories_set_us_free?language=en.

2. **"IF I EXAMINE SOMETHING, IT'S LESS SCARY":** *Joan Didion: The Center Will Not Hold*, directed by Griffin Dunne (Netflix, 2017), Netflix.

3. **SHAME IS HIGHLY CORRELATED WITH SELF-DESTRUCTIVE BEHAVIORS:** Kate Sheehy et al., "An Examination of the Relationship Between Shame, Guilt and Self-Harm: A Systematic Review and Meta-Analysis," *Clinical Psychology Review* 73 (November 1, 2019): 101779, https://doi.org/10.1016/j.cpr .2019.101779; Amy Y. Cameron, M. Tracie Shea, and Alyson B. Randall, "Acute Shame Predicts Urges for Suicide but Not for Substance Use in a Veteran Population," *Suicide and Life Threatening Behavior* 50, no. 1 (September 16, 2019): 292–99, https://doi.org/10.1111/sltb.12588; Diana-Mirela Nechita, Samuel Bud, and Daniel David, "Shame and Eating Disorders Symptoms: A Meta-Analysis," *International Journal of Eating Disorders* 54, no. 11 (July 24, 2021): 1899–945, https://doi.org/10.1002/eat.23583.

4. **AND EXTERNALIZING BEHAVIORS INCLUDING:** Jac Brown, "Shame and Domestic Violence: Treatment Perspectives for Perpetrators from Self Psychology and Affect Theory," *Sexual and Relationship Therapy* 19, no. 1 (February 1, 2004): 39–56, https://doi.org/10.1080/14681990410001640826; Patrizia Velotti, Jeff Elison, and Carlo Garofalo, "Shame and Aggression: Different Trajectories and Implications," *Aggression and Violent Behavior* 19, no. 4 (July 1, 2014): 454–61, https://doi.org/10.1016/j.avb.2014.04.011; Jonathan Fast, *Beyond Bullying: Breaking the Cycle of Shame, Bullying, and Violence* (Oxford, UK: Oxford University Press, 2016).

5. **IN THE DEVELOPMENT OF PERSONALITY TRAITS LIKE NARCISSISM AND EVEN PSYCHOPATHY:** Kathrin Ritter et al., "Shame in Patients with Narcissistic Personality Disorder," *Psychiatry Research* 215, no. 2 (February 1, 2014): 429–37, https://doi.org/10.1016/j.psychres.2013.11.019; Carlo Garofalo and Patrizia Velotti, "Shame Coping and Psychopathy: A Replication and Extension in a Sample of Male Incarcerated Offenders," *Journal of Criminal Justice* 76 (September 1, 2021): 101845, https://doi.org/10.1016/j.jcrimjus .2021.101845.

6. **IN THE WORDS OF KARL MARX:** Karl Marx to Arnold Ruge, March 1843, Mark and Engels Internet Archive: Letters, https://www.marxists.org /archive/marx/works/1843/letters/43_03-alt.htm.

7. **LINEHAN WROTE A CHAPTER ON VALIDATION:** Linehan, "Validation and Psychotherapy," 353–92.

8. **SHOW A SPIKE IN DOPAMINE AND AN INCREASED DESIRE TO USE:** Nora D. Volkow et al., "Dopamine in Drug Abuse and Addiction," *Archives of Neurology* 64, no. 11 (November 1, 2007): 1575, https://doi.org/10.1001/archneur .64.11.1575.

9. **MARTIN LUTHER KING JR. SAID:** Posted by Gabe Gentry, "Martin Luther King, Jr.—Where Do We Go from Here," YouTube, August 26, 2009, https://www .youtube.com/watch?v=GHJQCzv3dko.

10. **YOU'LL FIND IT DIFFICULT TO SLEEP:** Sergio González et al., "Circadian-Related Heteromerization of Adrenergic and Dopamine D4 Receptors Modulates Melatonin Synthesis and Release in the Pineal Gland," *PLOS Biology* 10, no. 6 (June 19, 2012): e1001347, https://doi.org/10.1371/journal .pbio.1001347.

CHAPTER 9: EQUALIZE—THE "ANYONE IN YOUR SHOES WOULD DO THE SAME" SKILL

1. **REQUIRES A HIGHER LEVEL OF COGNITIVE PROCESSING:** For a review of the visualization and cognitive processing research, see Christine D. Wilson-Mendenhall, John P. Dunne, and Richard J. Davidson, "Visualizing Compassion: Episodic Simulation as Contemplative Practice," *Mindfulness*, March 4, 2022, https://doi.org/10.1007/s12671-022-01842-6.

2. **GOLDEN RULE ARGUMENT:** "Golden Rule Argument," Legal Information Institute, accessed May 13, 2023, https://www.law.cornell.edu/wex/golden _rule_argument.

3. **"SOMEONE MUST HAVE BEEN":** Franz Kafka, *The Trial: Introduction by George Steiner* (London: Everyman's Library, 1992).

4. **"AN UNBELIEVABLE STORY OF RAPE":** T. Christian Miller and Ken Armstrong, "An Unbelievable Story of Rape," *ProPublica*, February 29, 2020, https:// www.propublica.org/article/false-rape-accusations-an-unbelievable -story.

5. **PULITZER PRIZE:** Pulitzer Prize Board, "Explanatory Reporting," Winners by Category, accessed April 30, 2023, https://www.pulitzer.org/prize-winners -by-category/207.

6. **SEVERAL DAYS LATER:** Miller and Armstrong, "An Unbelievable Story."

CHAPTER 10: PROPOSE—HOW TO READ MINDS

1. **EQ CAN BE IMPROVED:** Raquel Gilar-Corbi, Bárbara Yadira García Sánchez, and Juan Luis Castejón, "Can Emotional Intelligence Be Improved? A Randomized Experimental Study of a Business-Oriented EI Training Program for Senior Managers," *PLOS One* 14, no. 10 (October 23, 2019): e0224254, https://doi.org/10.1371/journal.pone.0224254; Nicholas Clarke, "The Impact of a Training Programme Designed to Target the Emotional Intelligence Abilities of Project Managers," *International Journal of Project Management* 28, no. 5 (July 1, 2010): 461–68, https://doi.org/10.1016/j.ij proman.2009.08.004.

2. **IN AN EPISODE TITLED "ROM-COM":** Elna Baker and Michelle Buteau, "638: Rom-Com, Act Two," February 9, 2018, in *This American Life*, produced by WBEZ, podcast, https://www.thisamericanlife.org/638/rom-com/act-two-23.

3. **INTERVIEWED THE FORMER DUCHESS OF SUSSEX:** Prince Harry and Meghan Markle, interview by Oprah Winfrey, *Oprah with Meghan and Harry*, CBS, March 7, 2021.

4. **BABE RUTH HAD AN IMPRESSIVE BATTING AVERAGE:** Shirley Povich, "Legend, Truth Mix with Ruth: 100th Anniversary of Babe's Birth," *The Washington Post*, February 5, 1995, https://www.washingtonpost.com/wp-srv/sports/longterm/general/povich/launch/ruth1.htm.

5. **PAUL EKMAN DEFINES MICRO EXPRESSIONS AS:** Paul Ekman Group, "Micro Expressions," Paul Ekman Group, accessed August 3, 2022, https://www.paulekman.com/resources/micro-expressions.

6. **"INVOLUNTARY EMOTIONAL LEAKAGE":** Paul Ekman Group, "Micro Expressions."

CHAPTER 11: TAKE ACTION—WHEN WORDS AREN'T ENOUGH

1. **IN A RARE INTERVIEW WITH ABC NEWS:** President Volodymyr Zelenskyy, interview by David Muir, *ABC World News Tonight*, ABC, March 7, 2022.

CHAPTER 12: EMOTE—MY ADVICE FOR JIMMY KIMMEL

1. **JON STEWART DELIVERED AN IMPASSIONED SPEECH:** ABC News, "Jon Stewart Slams Congress Over Benefits for 9/11 Responders," YouTube, June 11, 2019, https://www.youtube.com/watch?v=_uYpDC3SRpM&t=2s.

2. **AS NELSON MANDELA IS OFTEN QUOTED:** Nelson Mandela, *Nelson Mandela by Himself* (New York: Macmillan, 2011), 144.

3. **KIMMEL WENT ON AIR TO SHARE HIS EXPERIENCE:** *Jimmy Kimmel Live!*, created by Jimmy Kimmel, season 15, episode 57, aired May 1, 2022, on ABC.

CHAPTER 13: DISCLOSE—THE POWER OF ME, TOO

1. **IN 2021, MEHMET ÜMIT NECEF:** Mehmet Ümit Necef, "Research Note: Former Extremist Interviews Current Extremist: Self-Disclosure and Emotional Engagement in Terrorism Studies," *Studies in Conflict and Terrorism* 44, no. 1 (July 30, 2020): 74–92, https://doi.org/10.1080/1057610x.2020.1799516.

2. **"EMPTY HOLE INSIDE OF ME":** Necef, "Former Extremist Interviews Current Extremist," 77.

3. **NECEF WROTE: "HE IS TALKING AS I DID":** Necef, "Former Extremist Interviews Current Extremist," 78.

4. **ACCORDING TO NECEF, "MY SELF-DISCLOSURE":** Necef, "Former Extremist Interviews Current Extremist," 79–80.

5. **CIFTCI WAS NO LONGER MY 'RESEARCH OBJECT':** Necef, "Former Extremist Interviews Current Extremist," 80.

6. **AS BROWN PUTS IT:** Brené Brown, *Atlas of the Heart* (New York: Random House, 2021), 137.

7. **BROWN DEFINES SHAME AS:** Brown, *Atlas of the Heart*, 137.

8. **BURIED IN ARTICLES ON PSYCHOTHERAPY:** Jennifer R. Henretty and Heidi M. Levitt, "The Role of Therapist Self-Disclosure in Psychotherapy: A Qualitative Review," *Clinical Psychology Review* 30, no. 1 (February 1, 2010): 63–77, https://doi.org/10.1016/j.cpr.2009.09.004.

9. **GERMAN SOCIOLOGIST GEORG SIMMEL SAID:** Georg Simmel, "The Secret and the Secret Society," in *The Sociology of Georg Simmel*, ed. Kurt H. Wolff (Glencoe, IL: Free Press, 1950), 307.

CHAPTER 14: CH, CH, CH, CHANGES—BEHAVIORAL CHANGE STRATEGIES

1. **PARENT MANAGEMENT TRAINING:** Alan E. Kazdin, *Parent Management Training: Treatment for Oppositional, Aggressive, and Antisocial Behavior in Children and Adolescents* (Oxford, UK: Oxford University Press, 2005).

CHAPTER 15: RAISING EMOTIONALLY INTELLIGENT CHILDREN—VALIDATION AND PARENTING

1. **CASES OF ACTUAL ABUSE ASIDE:** Alan E. Kazdin and Carlo Rotella, *The Kazdin Method for Parenting the Defiant Child: With No Pills, No Therapy, No Contest of Wills* (Boston: Houghton Mifflin Harcourt, 2009).

2. **EMOTIONAL INVALIDATION DURING PARENT-CHILD CONFLICTS:** Sheila E. Crowell et al., "Mechanisms of Contextual Risk for Adolescent Self-Injury: Invalidation and Conflict Escalation in Mother–Child Interactions," *Journal of Clinical Child and Adolescent Psychology* 42, no. 4 (July 1, 2013): 467–80, https://doi.org/10.1080/15374416.2013.785360; Chad E. Shenk and Alan E. Fruzzetti, "Parental Validating and Invalidating Responses and Adolescent Psychological Functioning," *The Family Journal* 22, no. 1 (June 20, 2013): 43–48, https://doi.org/10.1177/1066480713490900.

3. **CHILDREN ARE MORE LIKELY TO BECOME DYSREGULATED:** Shenk and Fruzzetti, "Parental Validating and Invalidating"; Elizabeth L. Krause, Tamar Mendelson, and Thomas J. Lynch, "Childhood Emotional Invalidation and Adult Psychological Distress: The Mediating Role of Emotional Inhibition," *Child Abuse and Neglect* 27, no. 2 (February 1, 2003): 199–213, https://doi.org/10.1016/s0145-2134(02)00536-7.

4. **EMOTIONAL INVALIDATION DURING PARENT-CHILD CONFLICTS AND SUBSEQUENT SELF-HARM:** Molly Adrian et al., "Parental Validation and Invalidation Predict Adolescent Self-Harm," *Professional Psychology: Research and Practice* 49, no. 4 (August 1, 2018): 274–81, https://doi.org/10.1037/pro0000200.

5. **ATTENTION AND VALIDATION ARE LIKELY TO FURTHER DYSREGULATE THEM:** Nirbhay N. Singh, Bethany A. Marcus, and Ashvind N. Singh, "Differential Attention," in *Encyclopedia of Psychotherapy*, eds. Michel Hersen

and William Sledge (Philadelphia: Elsevier Science USA, 2002), 629–32; Thomas Sajwaj and Anneal Dillon, "Complexities of an 'Elementary' Behavior Modification Procedure: Differential Adult Attention Used for Children's Behavior Disorders," in *New Developments in Behavioral Research: Theory, Method, and Application*, 1st ed., eds. Barbara C. Etzel, Judith M. LeBlanc, and Donald M. Baer (Oxfordshire, UK: Routledge, 1977).

CHAPTER 16: THE UNIVERSAL LOVE LANGUAGE—VALIDATION IN INTIMATE RELATIONSHIPS

1. **NEGATIVE SENTIMENT OVERRIDE (NSO):** John M. Gottman, Carrie Cole, and Donald L. Cole. "Negative Sentiment Override in Couples and Families," in *Encyclopedia of Couple and Family Therapy*, eds. Jay L. Lebow, Anthony L. Chambers, and Douglas C. Breunlin (Berlin: Springer, 2019), 2019–22.

2. **COUPLES WHO VALIDATE EACH OTHER DURING CONFLICT:** Dean M. Busby and Thomas B. Holman, "Perceived Match or Mismatch on the Gottman Conflict Styles: Associations with Relationship Outcome Variables," *Family Process* 48, no. 4 (December 1, 2009): 531–45, https://doi.org/10.1111/j.1545-5300.2009.01300.x.

3. **ACCORDING TO JOHN GOTTMAN, THE NONVERBALS AND BASIC *MM-HMMS*:** John M. Gottman, "The Roles of Conflict Engagement, Escalation, and Avoidance in Marital Interaction: A Longitudinal View of Five Types of Couples," *Journal of Consulting and Clinical Psychology* 61, no. 1 (January 1, 1993): 6–15, https://doi.org/10.1037/0022-006x.61.1.6.

4. **RESEARCH SHOWS THAT A 5:1 RATIO:** John M. Gottman and Julie S. Gottman, "Gottman Method Couple Therapy," *Clinical Handbook of Couple Therapy*, 4th ed., ed. Alan S. Gurman (New York: Guilford Press, 2008), 138–64.

5. **THE "FOUR HORSEMEN OF THE APOCALYPSE":** John M. Gottman, *The Marriage Clinic: A Scientifically Based Marital Therapy* (New York: W. W. Norton & Company, 1999).

CHAPTER 17: VALIDATE LIKE A BOSS—VALIDATION AT WORK

1. **WHEN MANAGER MATT SAKAGUCHI:** Charles Duhigg, "What Google Learned from Its Quest to Build the Perfect Team," *New York Times Magazine*, February 25, 2016, https://www.nytimes.com/2016/02/28/magazine/what-google-learned-from-its-quest-to-build-the-perfect-team.html.

2. **"MY GOAL WITH THAT EXERCISE":** Matt Sakaguchi, interviewed by the Tory Burch Foundation, "What Sets Effective Teams Apart," accessed July 24, 2023, https://www.toryburchfoundation.org/resources/build-my-team/what-sets-effective-teams-apart.

3. **IN HER BOOK *THE FEARLESS ORGANIZATION*:** Amy C. Edmondson, *The Fearless Organization: Creating Psychological Safety in the Workplace for Learning, Innovation, and Growth* (Hoboken, NJ: John Wiley & Sons, 2019), xvi.

4. **PSYCHOLOGICAL SAFETY WAS FAR AND AWAY THE MOST IMPORTANT:** "Google's Project Aristotle," Re: Work with Google, Alphabet Inc., accessed July 25, 2023, https://rework.withgoogle.com/print/guides/5721312655835136.

5. **STUDIES IN INDUSTRIES RANGING FROM HEALTH CARE TO MANUFACTURING:** Amy C. Edmondson and Zhike Lei, "Psychological Safety: The History, Renaissance, and Future of an Interpersonal Construct," *Annual Review of Organizational Psychology and Organizational Behavior* 1, no. 1 (March 21, 2014): 23–43, https://doi.org/10.1146/annurev-orgpsych-031413 -091305.

6. **ACCORDING TO A 2017 GALLUP POLL:** Gallup, *State of the American Workplace Report* (Gallup, 2017), accessed March 1, 2023, https://www.gallup.com /workplace/238085/state-american-workplace-rep ort-2017.aspx.

7. **A SEPARATE POLL CONDUCTED BY CATALYST:** Catalyst and Edelman Intelligence, *The Impact of COVID-19 on Workplace Inclusion Survey* (Catalyst, 2020), accessed March 1, 2023, https://www.catalyst.org/research/work place-inclusion-covid-19.

8. **A STUDY OF MORE THAN FIFTEEN HUNDRED EMPLOYEES:** Dale Carnegie and Associates, Inc., *What Drives Employee Engagement and Why It Matters: Dale Carnegie Training White Paper* (Dale Carnegie and Associates, Inc., 2012).

9. **IN ANOTHER SURVEY OF MORE THAN NINE THOUSAND EMPLOYEES:** SHRM, *Global Culture Research Report* (SHRM, 2022), accessed February 3, 2023, https://www.shrm.org/hr-today/trends-and-forecasting/research-and -surveys/Documents/SHRM%202022%20Global%20Culture%20 Report.pdf.

10. **A STUDY OF MORE THAN TWENTY THOUSAND STUDENTS ACROSS THIRTY-FOUR DIFFERENT COLLEGES:** Sylvia Hurtado, Adriana Ruiz Alvarado, and Chelsea Guillermo-Wann, "Creating Inclusive Environments: The Mediating Effect of Faculty and Staff Validation on the Relationship of Discrimination /Bias to Students' Sense of Belonging," *Journal Committed to Social Change on Race and Ethnicity* 1, no. 1 (December 6, 2018): 59–81, https://doi.org/10 .15763/issn.2642-2387.2015.1.1.59-81.

11. **"THE VALIDATING EXPERIENCES CAN REINFORCE SELF-WORTH":** Hurtado, Ruiz Alvarado, and Guillermo-Wann, "Creating Inclusive Environments," 74.

12. **MANAGERS WITH STRONG INTERPERSONAL SKILLS:** Casey Mulqueen, Amy Kahn, and J. Stephen Kirkpatrick, "Managers' Interpersonal Skills and Their Role in Achieving Organizational Diversity and Inclusiveness," *Journal of Psychological Issues in Organizational Culture* 3, no. 3 (October 1, 2012): 48–58, https://doi.org/10.1002/jpoc.21062.

13. **"AN OUNCE OF GENUINE, OPEN-MINDED ACCEPTANCE":** Mulqueen, Kahn, and Kirkpatrick, "Managers' Interpersonal Skills," 49.

CHAPTER 18: EVERYBODY HURTS—SELF-VALIDATION

1.   **THE LYRICS FROM A DAVE MATTHEWS BAND SONG:** Dave Matthews Band, "Typical Situation," by Dave Matthews, recorded July 1994, track 5 on *Under the Table and Dreaming*, RCA, compact disc.

2.   **PEOPLE DEVELOP THESE BELIEFS IN RESPONSE TO PAINFUL EXPERIENCES IN CHILDHOOD:** Judith S. Beck, *Cognitive Therapy for Challenging Problems: What to Do When the Basics Don't Work* (New York: Guilford Press, 2011).

3.   **RESEARCH SUGGESTS THAT THE INVALIDATING BELIEFS:** Flávio Osmo et al., "The Negative Core Beliefs Inventory: Development and Psychometric Properties," *Journal of Cognitive Psychotherapy* 32, no. 1 (April 1, 2018): 67–84, https://doi.org/10.1891/0889-8391.32.1.67.

4.   **STUDIES HAVE SHOWN THAT:** Kristin D. Neff, Stephanie S. Rude, and Kristin L. Kirkpatrick, "An Examination of Self-Compassion in Relation to Positive Psychological Functioning and Personality Traits," *Journal of Research in Personality* 41, no. 4 (August 1, 2007): 908–16, https://doi.org/10.1016/j.jrp.2006.08.002.

5.   **SELF-VALIDATORS ALSO REPORT INCREASED MOTIVATION TO REPAIR:** Mark R. Leary et al., "Self-Compassion and Reactions to Unpleasant Self-Relevant Events: The Implications of Treating Oneself Kindly," *Journal of Personality and Social Psychology* 92, no. 5 (May 1, 2007): 887–904, https://doi.org/10.1037/0022-3514.92.5.887; Juliana G. Breines and Serena Chen, "Self-Compassion Increases Self-Improvement Motivation," *Personality and Social Psychology Bulletin* 38, no. 9 (May 29, 2012): 1133–43, https://doi.org/10.1177/0146167212445599.

6.   **THE APPROACH I DEVELOPED:** Germer and Neff, *The Mindful Self-Compassion Workbook*; Linehan, *DBT Skills Training*.

7.   **COMPASSION IS A SUBSET OF EMPATHY:** Edwin Rutsch, "Paul Ekman Talks Empathy with Edwin Rutsch," YouTube, May 10, 2011, https://www.youtube.com/watch?v=3i1QFv_PtqM.

8.   **THE MORE ONE FORGETS HIMSELF:** Viktor Emil Frankl, *Man's Search for Meaning*, 110. (Boston: Beacon Press, 1959). Originally published in 1946 as *Ein Psycholog erlebt das Konzentrationslager*.

9.   **YOU AND ME:** Ada Limón, "We Are Surprised," in *Bright Dead Things* (Minneapolis: Milkweed Editions, 2015).

10.   **ACCEPTANCE IS THE FIRST STEP:** "MARSHA LINEHAN: How She Learned Radical Acceptance," YouTube, April 14, 2017, https://www.youtube.com/watch?v=f8iNYY7YV04.

EPILOGUE

1. **TO QUOTE DELGAUDIO:** Sam Schube, "Derek DelGaudio's Genre-Bending Magic Show Will Make You Feel Things," *GQ*, July 16, 2018, https://www.gq.com/story/derek-delgaudio-magician-profile.

2. **TO QUOTE RENOWNED SOCIAL PSYCHOLOGIST:** Mark R. Leary and Ashley Batts Allen, "Belonging Motivation: Establishing, Maintaining, and Repairing Relational Value," in *Social Motivation*, ed. David Dunning (New York: Psychology Press, 2011), 37–55.

INDEX

5:1 ratio of positivity to negativity during
conflicts, 235
9/11 Victim Compensation Fund (VCF)
testimony example of validation
skills, 173–75

A
abuse, 118
academic validation, 249
acceptance
Carl Rogers' theories about, 60–61
as a catalyst for change, 13–14, 267
radical acceptance, 14–15
strategies, 14
ACCEPTED acronym of the eight skills in
the Validation Ladder, 74–75
Attend, 81–97
Copy, 99–112
Contextualize, 113–24
Equalize, 125–39
Propose, 141–56
Take Action, 157–71
Emote, 173–88
Disclose, 189–202
addiction, 120, 195
Adler, Marie, 132–33
the *A Game*, 90–91, 145
agreement, 49–51
Alison, Laurence and Emily, 28–29
apologies, 226
approval, 51
Attend skill of the Validation Ladder
the *A Game*, 90–91, 145
defined, 85
as depicted in Derek DelGaudio's *In
and Of Itself*, 81–85

forging connections by showing up,
85–86
how to demonstrate the, 87–93
mistakes and solutions, 93–95
showing interest, 86–87
summary, 95–96
synonymous terms, 85n
tips for practicing the, 96–97
when self-validating, 255–57
when to use the, 93
attention, paying, 41–42
authenticity, 45, 74
autism spectrum conditions (ASC), 106n

B
Baaren, Rick B. van, 100
Baker, Elna, 143–45, 147n
behavior
behavioral intentions, 31
changes when the subject knows
they're being observed, 85
culturally appropriate, 47
defined, 211
determining the validity of, 47–48
effect of past circumstances on
current, 119–20
Emoting nonverbal, 177–79, 188
immediacy behaviors ("the Big Four"),
87–88, 177
positive effects of validation on
behavior change, 4, 32–33
beliefs, invalidating strongly held, 137
Biden, Joe, 160
borderline personality disorder (BPD),
55–56
boundary-crossing, 199–200

Brown, Brené, 193, 194
Building a Life Worth Living (Linehan), 20, 59
Buteau, Michelle, 143–45, 147n

C
case studies
Dev (estrangement from her daughter), 23–26, 28, 30
Ella (empathy), 43–44, 67
garbage bin situation, 50–51
Jeff (contextualizing a behavior issue), 113–14
Juanita and John (parenting responsibilities), 231–32, 233
Keith (validating his daughter), 216–17
Lou (perfectionism needing Equalizing), 134–35
Marcia and Clara (intimacy issues), 231, 233, 234
Michael (insensitive comments at work), 245–46
obsessive-compulsive disorder (OCD) client with transportation issues, 164–65, 167
Pam and Dwight (workplace attitude conversation), 244, 246
Sam (bathroom signage), 166, 167
Sergey and Melinda (door slamming disagreement), 236–37
terminated employee sharing vulnerable emotions, 181–82
celebrity talk show hosts and their natural validation skills, 71–72, 77, 187–88
the chameleon effect, 105–07
change strategies
author's work with a feral cat, 205–11
classical conditioning, 207
extinction, 210
modeling, 212
negative reinforcement, 209–10
operant conditioning, 207
positive reinforcement, 12, 32–34, 209
problem-solving, 212–13
shaping, 208–09, 231
ubiquity of, 12

children, validating
apologies, 226
debriefs, 224–26
discipline *vs.* conflict resolution, 224–27
dysregulation, 221–22, 223
emotional invalidation of, 221–24
Golden Snitch idea, 217–20
the most validating skills to use with, 217
reinforcing behavior, 219–20
summary points to remember, 227
Ciftci, Enes, 191–92
communication
author's experiences with validation, 129–31
idea dial concept, 146–49
compassion
self-compassion, 4, 35
conditioning
classical, 207
defined, 119–20
operant, 207
shaping, 208–09
conflict
Copy skill of the Validation Ladder as a cure for, 107–10
discipline *vs.* conflict resolution, 224–27
in intimate relationships, 234–37
positive effects of validation on, 3, 28–30
connections, forging
Craig Foster and the octopus example, 85–86
in daily life, 86
through the highest levels of validation, 183
Contextualize skill of the Validation Ladder
author's friend's experiences, 113–14
challenging "shoulds," 116
defined, 114
disorders that conflict with personal goals, 121–22
misinformation, 120–21
the role of fear, 117–19, 248
summary, 122–23

tips for practicing the, 123–24
understanding the logical reasoning
that led to someone's reaction,
114–15
validating problem behavior in
specific contexts, 119–22
when self-validating, 258–59
control, losing, 184–85, 186
the Conversation Tell, 153–54
Copy skill of the Validation Ladder
author's experiences using, 102–04
the chameleon effect, 105–07
as a cure for conflict, 107–10
defined, 99
in a relaxed manner, 110–11
research about the effectiveness of
the, 100–02
summary, 111–12
tips for practicing the, 112
validating benefits of the, 105–07
when self-validating, 257–58
when speaking with young
children, 111
couples therapy, 107–08
cultural norms regarding eye
contact, 87n
customer relations, 29

D
debriefs, 224–26
DelGaudio, Derek, 81–85, 88, 92–93, 100
depression
author's experiences with major
depressive disorder, 2, 193–94
exercise as a treatment for, 11n
Dev case study (estrangement from her
daughter), 23–26, 28, 30
Dialectical Behavior Therapy (DBT),
13–15, 17–18, 58–59, 62–65
Didion, Joan, 117
diminishing someone's experience, 136
discipline *vs.* conflict resolution,
224–27
Disclose skill of the Validation Ladder
avoiding sharing an unresolved
experience, 200–01
boundary-crossing, 199–200
defined, 190

degrees of disclosure, 192–95
effectiveness and tolerance of
disclosed information, 196
the invalidation of shame, 193–95
losing focus, 197–99
mistakes and solutions, 195–201
MS example of the power of the,
189, 195
Necef and Ciftci extremist behavior
example of the power of the,
191–92
overshadowing the client, 196–97
to show relatability, 195
summary, 201
tips for practicing the, 202
discrimination, 101–02, 249
disorders that conflict with personal
goals, 121–22
diversity and inclusion, 247–49
dysregulation, 221–22, 223

E
Edmondson, Amy, 240–41
Ekman, Paul, 153–54
Ella case study (empathy), 43–44, 67
Emote skill of the Validation Ladder
audio and visual examples of the,
187–88
author's experiences with the, 176,
184–85
in daily life, 176–77
defined, 175
holding back emotions, 182–83
implying emotions, 179–80
Jon Stewart's Congressional testimony
about 9/11 first responders,
173–75, 177–78, 179
labeling emotions, 179
losing control of one's emotions,
184–85, 186
mistakes and solutions, 183–86
nonverbal behavior, 177–79, 188
playing it cool when sharing emotions,
181–82
summary, 186–87
tips for practicing the, 187–88
when self-validating, 261–62
emotional intelligence (EQ), 143, 152

emotions
  "emotional leakage," 153–54
  holding back, 182–83
  implying, 179–80
  labeling, 179
  negative, 223
  playing it cool when sharing, 181–82
  proportionate, 48–49
  validity of, 48–49, 163n, 221–24
  vulnerable, 181–82
empathy
  compared to sympathy, 43–45
  Golden Rule approach, 128–29, 259–60
  skill set of the Validation Ladder,
    73–74, 78
Equalize skill of the Validation Ladder
  author's family hiking experience,
    125–27
  the Caroline Qualifier, 130–31, 136–37,
    138–39
  critical times for implementing the,
    131–36
  defined, 127
  mistakes and solutions, 136–37
  summary, 137–38
  third-person comparison, 130
  tips for practicing the, 138–39
  using logical reasoning and
    communication, 128–31
  when self-validating, 259–60
exercise as a treatment for depression, 11n
eye contact, 87–88, 94

F
facial expressions, 152–53
fear, 117–19, 248
The Fearless Organization (Edmondson),
  240–41
feedback, 178–79, 222–23
Fights, Games, and Debates (Rapoport),
  109–10
Fleck, Caroline
  behavioral change work with a feral
    cat, 205–11
  breast cancer experiences, 269–71,
    272–73
  the Caroline Qualifier, 130–31, 136–37,
    138–39

childhood sensitivity, 1–2
communicating with her father, 179–80
experiences treating an obsessive-
  compulsive disorder (OCD) client,
  164–65, 167
experiences treating a schizophrenic
  client, 46
experiences treating a suicidal client,
  9–11, 145–46
family hiking experience example of
  Equalizing, 125–27
garage cleaning story, 32–33
interactions with Havana, 32–33, 34,
  125–27, 129–30, 161, 163, 210–11,
  218–19
interactions with Mat, 102–04, 148–49
losing control while treating the
  mother of a suicidal teen, 184–85
major depressive disorder
  experiences, 2, 193–94
multiple sclerosis (MS) diagnosis and
  effects, 55–59, 66, 189, 195, 251
postpartum dinner help experiences,
  167–68
tendency to copy others' accents, 105
thoughts about suffering, 66–67
writing experiences, 244–45, 246,
  264–67
focus, losing, 197–99
Foster, Craig, 85–86
Frankl, Viktor, 65–66

G
Gamache Martin, Christina, 30–31
garbage bin situation case study, 50–51
gender issues
  pervasive invalidation, 36
Germer, Christopher, 35
Golden Rule approach, 128–29, 259–60
Golden Snitch idea, 217–20
Gotman-Rapoport Intervention
  ("Rapoport"), 108–10
Gottman, John, 107–10, 235
guilt and shame, 118–19, 193–95, 226

H
Hanh, Thich Nhat, 65–66
Harvard Study of Adult Development, 23n

Havana (author's daughter)
  behavior regulation, 210–11
  family hiking experience example of
    Equalizing, 125–27
  garage cleaning story, 32–33
  hair brushing assistance, 161
  honesty Golden Snitch moment,
    218–19
  nightmare experience, 111
  playing with her mother when sick, 34
  skiing experiences, 163
  spelling test disappointment, 52–53
hypotheses *vs.* assumptions, 124

I
idea dial concept, 146–49
identity invalidation, 35–36
immediacy behaviors, 87–88
implying emotions, 179–80
In and Of Itself (film), 81–85
influence
  attempting to change others' behavior,
    11–12
  positive effects of validation on, 3–4,
    30–32
intensity, 94
intimate relationships
  5:1 ratio of positivity to negativity
    during conflicts, 235
  avoiding criticism or invalidation,
    232–34
  conflict management, 234–37
  examples of couples' issues, 231–34
  negative sentiment override (NSO),
    230–31
  punishment, 229–33, 237
  summary, 237
  using the principles of change, 229–30
invalidation, 25, 34–36, 212, 221–24,
  253–54

J
Jeff case study (contextualizing a
  behavior issue), 113–14
Jimmy Kimmel Live! (TV show), 182
Josef K. in *The Trial,* 131–32
Journal of Interpersonal Violence (journal),
  31–32

Juanita and John case study
  (parenting responsibilities),
    231–32, 233
judgment, 121

K
Kabat-Zinn, Jon, 16, 18
Kafka, Franz, 131–32
Kazdin, Alan, 210
Keith case study (validating his
  daughter), 216–17
"kernel of truth," searching for the,
  45–46, 63
Kimmel, Jimmy, 182
King, Martin Luther, Jr., 121

L
labeling emotions, 179
language choices, 179–80
learning
  through repetition, 75
  by watching others, 76
Leary, Mark, 274
Linehan, Marsha
  acceptance work, 61–62
  Dialectical Behavior Therapy (DBT),
    13–15, 17–18, 58–59, 62–65
  interactions with the author, 55, 58–59,
    66–67
  memoir, 20, 59
  studies in Zen Buddhism, 62
  validation work, 16–17, 18, 119
listening
  the *A Game,* 90–91, 145
  asking questions and commenting,
    91–93
  engagement requirements for, 89
  validation as a way of increasing,
    31–32
logical reasoning
  default approach, 128
  Golden Rule approach, 128–29,
    259–60
  for using the Propose skill of the
    Validation Ladder, 143–46
loneliness, 68
Lou case study (perfectionism needing
  Equalizing), 134–35

M
major depressive disorder
author's experiences, 2, 193–94
the stigma of mental illness, 193–95
Mandela, Nelson, 180
manipulation, 214
Man's Search for Meaning (Frankl), 65–66
Marcia and Clara case study (intimacy issues), 231, 233, 234
Markle, Meghan, 147
Marx, Karl, 118
Mat (author's husband)
Copy skill conversation with the author, 102–04
family hiking experience example of Equalizing, 125–27
health conversations with the author, 148–49
Michael case study (insensitive comments at work), 245–46
micro expressions, 152–53
mindfulness
defined, 16
paying attention, 41–42
skill set of the Validation Ladder, 73–74, 78, 248–49
Mindfulness-Based Stress Reduction (MBSR), 16
The Mindful Self-Compassion Workbook (Neff and Germer), 35
misinformation, 120–21
Murthy, Vivek, 68
My Octopus Teacher (film), 85–86

N
Necef, Mehmet Ümit, 191–92
Neff, Kristin, 35
negative sentiment override (NSO), 230–31
negativity bias, 42–43, 230
nonverbal behaviors
Emoting, 177–79, 188
signs of validation, 152
"the Big Four," 87–88, 177

O
Obama, Barack, 20
obsessive-compulsive disorder (OCD)

client with transportation issues case study, 164–65, 167
Oprah (TV show), 77

P
Pam and Dwight case study (workplace attitude conversation), 244, 246
past circumstances and current behavior, 119–20
Perceived Partner Responsiveness (PPR), 27n
perfectionism, 133–36
positive reinforcement, 12, 32–34, 209
praise, 51, 242–43
problem-solving
as a change strategy, 212–13
vs. Taking Action, 158–59
vs. validation, 39–41, 52–53
Project Aristotle studies of high-performing teams, 239–41
Propose skill of the Validation Ladder
author's experiences using, 141–42, 150
the Conversation Tell, 153–54
defined, 141
idea dial concept, 146–49
mistakes, detecting and recovering from, 149–54
soulmate effect, 141–42, 145
summary, 154–55
tips for practicing the, 155–56
using logical reasoning and communication, 143–49
psychoanalysis, 61
psychological safety, 199–200, 240–41
punishment
of children, 220–24
in intimate relationships, 229–33, 237
self-punishment, 254
Putin, Vladimir, 86

Q
questions
To Act or Not to Act when considering Taking Action, 161–64
Attending questions *vs.* suggestions Proposed as questions, 147n

R
racial relations
   Copying research regarding implicit
      racism, 101–02
   diversity and inclusion, 247–49
   racial identity invalidation, 35
   students' feelings of belonging, 249
radical acceptance, 14–15
Rapoport, Anatol, 109
Rapoport (Gotman-Rapoport
   Intervention), 108–10
rapport, 29
relationships
   intimate, 229–37
   positive effects of validation on, 3,
      27–28
   and their effect on health and
      happiness, 23n
repetition, 75
rewards, 12, 32–34, 209
Rogers, Carl, 58–59, 60–61
Ruth, Babe, 149

S
Sakaguchi, Matt, 239–41
Sam (bathroom signage) case study,
   166, 167
self-compassion
   described, 35
   positive effects of validation on, 4
self-disclosure, 31
self-harm, 222
self-invalidation. See invalidation
self-punishment, 254
self-soothing, 262
self-validation
   as an exercise in self-compassion, 35
   author's experiences using, 270–72
   teaching, 36
   using the Validation Ladder skills,
      254–64, 265
sensitivity
   author's experiences, 1–2
   difficulties communicating feelings,
      44–45
September 11th Victim Compensation
   Fund (VCF) testimony example of
   validation skills, 173–75

Sergey and Melinda case study (door
   slamming disagreement), 236–37
shame and guilt, 118–19, 193–95, 226
shoulds, 116
Simmel, Georg, 202
Skinner, B. F., 12n, 61, 207n, 214
soulmate effect when using the Propose
   skill of the Validation Ladder,
      141–42, 145
Sparrow Baggins (author's cat), 205–11
speech patterns, modifying your, 92–93
Stewart, Jon, 173–75, 177–78, 179
suffering
   author's experiences, 66–67
   decreasing suffering by attending to
      others, 65
   finding meaning in, 59, 65–66
suicide
   author's experiences treating a
      suicidal client, 9–11, 145–46
   losing control while treating the
      mother of a suicidal teen, 184–85
sympathetic nervous system response,
   29–30
sympathy, 43

T
Take Action skill of the Validation Ladder
   To Act or Not to Act questions, 161–64
   alternatives to providing help, 169
   author's postpartum help experiences,
      167–68
   the busybodying mistake, 168–69
   compared to problem-solving, 158–59
   defined, 158
   similarity to other validation skills
      taught by Marsha Linehan, 158n
   summary, 170
   tips for practicing the, 170–71
   Ukraine-Russia situation, 157–58, 160
   when others cannot Take Action
      themselves, 160–67
   when self-validating, 262–64
   when someone hasn't asked you to
      intervene, 166–67
talking
   self-disclosure, 31
   validation as a way of increasing, 30–31

terminated employee sharing vulnerable emotions case study, 181–82
This American Life (podcast), 143–45
thoughts, validity of, 47
timing of conversations, 94–95
torture, 28–29
touch, 261
The Trial (Kafka), 131–32
trust, 30

U
Ukraine-Russia situation, 157–58, 160
"An Unbelievable Story of Rape" (article), 132–33
understanding
  defined, 42
  focusing on what's valid, 42–43
  skill set of the Validation Ladder, 73–74, 78

V
validation
  academic, 249
  asking for, 272–74
  defined, 16–17, 41
  invalidating strongly held beliefs, 137
  invalidation, 25, 34–36, 212, 221–24, 253–54
  the need for, 212, 213
  nonverbal signs of, 152
  positive changes from practicing, 3–5
  vs. praise, 242–43
  vs. problem-solving, 39–41, 52–53
  self-validation, 35, 36, 251–67
  skills, 19–20
  teaching, 75–76
  uses of, 18, 26, 53
  validating only what is valid, 45–49, 163
  as a way to influence behavior, 15
the Validation Ladder
  1—mindfulness skills, 73–74, 78, 248–49

2—understanding skills, 73–74, 78
3—empathy skills, 73–74, 78
ACCEPTED acronym of the eight skills in, 74–75
  Attend, 81–97
  Copy, 99–112
  Contextualize, 113–24
  Equalize, 125–39
  Propose, 141–56
  Take Action, 157–71
  Emote, 173–88
  Disclose, 189–202
cheat sheet, 275–76
diagram, 73
failing while practicing, 76–78
importance of position on, 79
skills to use when self-validating, 254–64
violence
  dating violence, 31–32
  pervasive invalidation as a contributor to, 36
vulnerability, 78

W
Winfrey, Oprah, 77, 147, 151
workplace validation
  diversity and inclusion, 247–49
  employee engagement, 243
  importance of psychological safety, 240–41
  Matt Sakaguchi's experiences, 239–41
  the need for, 242–43
  praise vs. validation, 242–43
  Project Aristotle studies of high-performing teams, 239–41
  reinforcing people at work, 243–47
  using mindfulness skills to understand others' experiences, 248–49

Z
Zelenskyy, Volodymyr, 157–58, 160